A TREATISE ON OBSTETRICS

DISORDERS OF PREGNANCY, PARTURITION AND LACTATION

JOHN C. PETERS, M.D.

B. JAIN PUBLISHERS (P) LTD.

Note from the Publishers

Any information given in this book is not intended to be taken as a replacement for medical advice. Any person with a condition requiring medical attention should consult a qualified practitioner or therapeutist.

A TREATISE ON OBSTETRICS

Reprint Edition: Jan. 2005

No part of this book may be reproduced, stored in a retrieval system or transmitted, in any form or by any means, mechanical, photocopying, recording or otherwise, without any prior written permission of the publishers.

© Copyright with the publishers.

Price: Rs. 55.00

Published by Kuldeep Jain for
B. Jain Publishers (P) Ltd.
1921, Street No. 10, Chuna Mandi,
Paharganj, New Delhi 110 055 (INDIA)
Phones: 2358 0800, 2358 1100, 2358 1300
Fax: 011-2358 0471; *Email:* bjain@vsnl.com
Website: www.bjainbooks.com

Printed in India by
J.J. Offset Printers
522, FIE, Patpar Ganj, Delhi - 110 092
Phones: 2216 9633, 2215 6128

ISBN: 81-7021-034-8

BOOK CODE: BJ-2416

INTRODUCTORY.

THIS is a valuable guide for Homœopathic profession for the treatment of "Diseases of Pregnancy, Parturition and Lactation", arranged with reference to well authenticated observations at the sick bed to facilitate and secure the selection of a suitable remedy.

In this book Dr. Peters begins with an unusually thorough discussion of the aspect of patient "Diseases of Married Female".

This work is indispensable to the students and practitioners of Homœopathy and highly interesting. It is hoped, this edition will meet with a wormer welcome and appreciation.

PUBLISHERS.

Calcutta, 5th May, 1973.

AUTHOR'S PREFACE.

THIS work is compiled and arranged upon the same plan as the Treatise on Disorders of Menstruation, lately published. I claim no unusual amount of knowledge or experience upon the subjects of which it treats; in fact it was undertaken as much for my own instruction as that of others. It is intended more especially for the junior medical practitioner, for experienced nurses, and for mothers. I have sought to avoid the confusing intricacy of complete and compendious treatises on Midwifery, and to escape the trifling pomposity of catch-penny popular works. The works of Cazeaux, Colombat, Murphy, Whitehead, Tilt, Ticknor, Tracy, Anderson, Churchill, Valleix, Vernois, Becquerel, Leadam, Croserio, and Williamson have been freely used, and the language of the respective authors has generally been adopted.

J. C. PETERS.

ON THE DISEASES

OF

PREGNANCY, PARTURITION, AND LACTATION,

ON MARRIAGE.

WE take it for granted that, in civilized countries, marriage only takes place between persons of proper age, and from the dictates of reason and personal affection. From 18 to 25 years of age may be considered the most proper period for females to contract marriage; from 25 to 30 years for males.

Interest, superstition, and still more unworthy motives, have, however, in all ages, led to earlier marriages. According to ROBERTON, marriages of interest were, perhaps, more abused in England, up to the year 1660, than in any other country; and that not always for the interest of the contracting female; but, on the contrary, frequently to her great detriment in person and estate. Then, almost all the property of the English realm was, by the policy of the laws, supposed to be granted by, dependent upon, or holden of some superior chief or lord; even wardship and marriage were under the control of these grasping freebooters. The right of wordship meant, that the lord had the guardianship of his tenant during his minority, by virtue of which right he had both the care of his person, and reserved to his own use the profit of the estate, except the word's sustenance and clothing, the amount of which lay much at the mercy of his lord. Further, by a gross abuse of this custom in England, this right of wardship was often, by the lord, assigned over to strangers; or it was put up to sale, or bequeathed by will, like any other kind of disposable property. But, besides the profit of the estate during the minority, the lord had another perquisite connected with his guardianship, viz., the right of disposing of his ward, whether male or female, in matrimony. If the lord did not make over or sell his right, he soon set about finding matches for his wards, either by uniting them, if that were thought advantageous, with members of his own family, or of the families of relatives, or by selling the marriage, *i.e.*, if the ward, for example, were a female, disposing of her hand to the best bidder, provided he was of suitable rank; for the law forbade disparagement. The marriage, in most of these cases, instead of being delayed to the period of legal consent for the female, which was 12 years, were often contracted at an age considerably earlier with a view to its being consummated when the parties should arrive at puberty, or before that period. But it often happened that the lord, instead of exercising the right of guardian, sold it to a stranger, one prompted by every pecuniary, or baser motive, to abuse the delicate and important trust of education; without any ties of blood or regard, to counteract the temptations of interest; or any sufficient authority to restrain him from yielding to their influence. Thus, william Bishop of Ely, gave 220 marks for the custody of Stephen de Beanchamp, and the right to marry him to whom he pleased: John, Earl of Lincoln, gave 3000 marks to have the marriage of Richard de Clare for the benefit of his eldest daughter, Mitilda, &c., &c. But the most curious thing, says ROBERTON, connected with the treatment of this species of property, is the extremely cool manner in which wards were bequeathed, along with ordinary goods and chattels; thus, Sir John Cornwallis, in his will (1554), after a very

MARRIAGE.

devout and pious exordium, says; I bequeath to my daughter, my wife's gown of black velvet; to my son Henry, my own gown of tawny taffeta; to my son Richard, my ward Margaret Lowthe, which I bought of my Lord of Norfolk, to marry her himself, if they will be so contented; but, if not, I will that he shall have the wardship and marriage of her, with all the advantages and profits. Sir Reginald Bray says, in his will: "Whereas, I have in my keeping Elizabeth and Agnes, daughters and heirs of Henry Lovell, Esq., I will that Elizabeth be married to one of my nephews, son to my brother, John Bray, and the said Agnes to another son of my said brother."

The dread of this unrighteous slaveship, that wardship and marriage, often operated with parents in marrying their children at a tender age. Thus, Maurice, 4th Lord of Berkeley, was knighted at 7, and married at 8 years old, to Elizabeth, daughter of Hugh, Lord Spencer, then but 8 years old. This early marriage prevented wardship, the payment of a large fine to the King, and assisted the party's own affairs with family interest and powerful connections. In fact, the Lords of Berkeley, some years ago, differed but little in their marriages from the customs of the most lascivious, depraved, and mercenary of savages, or slave-holders. The majority of the Berkeleys were contracted in marriage at 7 or 8 years of age, and in their family records more than a dozen instances occur of paternity before the age of 14. Throughout all England such precocity was once unblushingly encouraged, assimilating the people of a Christian country, in this revolting feature, to the Pagan inhabitants of the tropical regions.—ROBERTON.

GRAFTON, however, a faithful chronicler in the reign of Elizabeth, gives the following extremely curious display of humane and patriotic feeling:

"It is to be much lamented, that wards are brought and sold as commonly as are beasts; and marriages are made with them, that are many times very ungodly; for divers of them, being of young and tender years, are forced to judge by another man's affections, and to see with another man's eye, and to say yea with another man's tongue, and finally consent with another man's heart. For none of these senses be perfected to the parties in that minority, and so the election being unfree, and the years unripe, each of them, almost of necessity, must hate the other, whom yet they have had no judgment to love. And, certainly the common bargaining and selling of them is to be abhorred, for besides being stript out of almost all the property they have, they are handled, as the common saying is, like wards. Who seeth not, daily, what innumerable inconveniences, divorces, yea, and some murders, have proceeded from such marriages, or rather no marriages."—ROBERTON.

In some European countries, *late* marriages are enforced by law, and the laws against early and improvident marriages are extremely strict. In Wurtemberg, no man is allowed to marry, under the age of 25, unless permission has been especially obtained or purchased; in Saxony, a man liable to serve in the army, may not marry under 21; in Mecklenburg, men do not generally marry until 25 or 30, and the women not much earlier, etc. In Bavaria, the clergy are held responsible for the support of those poor persons whom they marry without permission of the authorities, besides being fined. In Norway, no one can marry until he has satisfied the clergyman that he is able to maintain a family. ROBERTON.

The consequences of these stringent laws are not always good; for illicit intercourse is almost necessasily at a premium, and it is a lamentable truth, that in the whole of South Germany, more illegitimate children are born, than legitimate.

With great show of justice, it is asserted, that a girl is hardly fit to receive attention in view of a future Marriage relation, before her 18th year; at which time her understanding and discrimination are fully awake to guide her to a proper selections. If she then has been sufficiently in the company of men, and has perhaps tried her heart and hand a little with a few innocent flirtations, she may be able, with her parent's assistance, to appreciate understandingly the character of those who approach her, and make a wise selection. It is his firm conviction, that the female constitution is only sufficiently consolidated and established at 21 years of age, to allow of Marriage, without injury to health and comfort. A few exceptions to this rule may be found, in which girls of 18 have acquired the mental and physical perfection, which the majority only attain some years later. But then some naively say, a young lady of proper age and health of body and mind, ought to marry as soon as she and her parents are firmly convinced that she has found a worthy partner; and no trifling cause should be allowed to divert her from the path of duty and happiness which nature intended her to follow and enjoy. No petty selfishness, no fear of hardships or troubles, should influence or agitate the mind to such an exent as suppress the kindlier feelings of her nature, at a time of life, when it is naturally the most capable of exciting and reciprocating love. They take this ground because it is also assumed that a greater degree of health generally attends wives and mothers, than those who remain unmarried.

CONCEPTION.

The monthly development of ovules or germs of future beings, in the ovaries of the female, has been sufficiently dwelt upon in my book upon the Disorders of Menstruation. (See pages 2 and 3). As a matter of course, the most proper period for conception, or fecundation, will be that immediately before or after the flow of the menses; in fact, RACIBORSKY has actually ascertained that conception took place a little before or after menstruation, in 15 females, all of whom could designate precisely the period of exposure. CAZEAUX truly says, it is very evident that everything seems admirably prepared at this period for the reproduction of the species; still he does not believe that the aptitude for fecundation in the human race is always limited to a few days, either preceding or following the menstrual periods; because he thinks that the excitement during intercourse may communicate itself to the ovarian vesicles, and cause changes in them altogether similar to those experienced at the menstrual period. Still, those persons who are anxious to increase their families, had better select the periods comprising a few days before and after the monthly period, as the most proper time for that purpose. While those, who for the various reasons of health, poverty, &c., are necessarily obliged to have as small a family as the exigencies of life will permit of, should at the very least exert self-control at these times.

CAZEAUX says, it is extremely difficult, if not impossible, to fix a precise period at which the fecundated ovule actually reaches the cavity of the womb; in fact, it is extremely probable that the time varies, and in the present records of science there is no proof that such ovules have seen in the uterus of a woman, prior to the 10th or 12th day after conception. This period coincides with of the formation and expulsion of the delicate decidual membrane or cast, which, according to POUCHET, is found in the cavity of the womb at every menstruation, even in virgins.

All these facts agree with the latest scientific assumption, that the periodical monthly returns of ovarian activity and congestion, tend to the growth, development, and expulsion from the ovaries into the womb, of the ovules or germs of future beings, one of which is sacrificed at each monthly period, unless conception take place; while the simultaneous periodic activity and congestion of the womb tends to the production of the envelopes or membranes, which should enshroud the

CONCEPTION.

germ, and if conception take place, to the proper supply of it with blood, and materials for growth and development. It is almost always desirable to ascertain the exact date of conception. CAZEAUX thinks that the woman is apt to experience an emotion of painful pleasure, and a shuddering, preceding from the spine, pain in the region of the navel, sometimes a sensation of motion in the abdomen, and uneasy feelings in the region of the hips, followed by languor, fatigue, and sleepiness, and the next day, by a sense of fullness, warmth, and heaviness in the abdomen. With the aid of some such signs, CAZEAUX says, that some females, especially those who have already had children, are able to distinguish a prolific intercourse; he has met with too many women who are thus adept, not to believe there is some truth in their assertions.

PREGNANCY.

This state commences at the instant of fecundation, and terminates with the expulsion of the child from its mother's body; it is supposed, on an average, to continue from 270 days, or 9 solar months, to 280 days, or 10 lunar months; some authors think the labor is particularly apt to set in at the exact time of what would be the 9th or 10th monthly period after the "suppression of Pregnancy." We will say a few words here on this point, as a woman scarcely imagines that she has conceived, before she begins to calculate when her Pregnancy, will probably end. We are sorry to say that there is a great variety in the length of gestation; there is, in fact, according to MERRIMAN, often a difference of 56 days between the two extremes of natural, but early delivery, and natural, but retarded labor; he thinks that nearly 5 per cent. of all women overrun the average term of 9 months, by as much as 10 or 12 days.

MERRIMAN has furnished a summary of 150 gestations,

in each of which he noted the precise day of the menses' last appearance. Of these,

5 women were delivered in the 37th week, *i.e.*, in from 252 to 259 days.

16 in the 38th week, or in from 262 to 266 days.

21	"	39th	"	"	"	267	"	273	"
46	"	40th	"	"	"	274	"	280	"
28	"	41st	"	"	"	281	"	287	"
18	"	42d	"	"	"	288	"	294	"
11	"	43d	"	"	"	295	"	301	"
5	"	44th	"	"	"	303	"	306	"

In my book, on the Disorders of Menstruation, it has been shown, (see pages 16, 17, 21, 22,) that the period of regular menstruation varies in many females; only from 61 to 71 per cent. following the 4-weekly, or lunar monthly, or 28 day type. Hence, if the time of delivery is a multiple of the menstrual period, those women who follow the 3-weekly menstrual type will probably have a delivery differing in time from that of those who follow the 4-weekly, or 6-weekly type.

Again, as many women conceive just before an expected menstrual period, which is then unexpectedly suppressed, they are apt to commence their calculation from the period before, and thus make their preparations for delivery, 2 or 3 weeks too early.

As soon as conception takes place, the consequent increased flow of blood towards the womb sensibly increases, first the volume of the uterine walls, and subsequently dilates their cavity. This increase of size and volume is also kept up and soon augmented by the deposit of some plastic and coagulable lymph, probably merely in increase of the delicate deciduous membrane, or cast, which we have seen is formed at each menstrual period; but long before the arrival of the impregnated ovule from the ovaries and fallopian tubes, a kind of pouch or vesicle has been formed in the womb for its reception, and to which ovologists have given the name of caducous membrane. As soon as the ovule has arrived in the womb, the uterus begins to develope, and its volume continues to increase until the end of Pregnancy; but this progression in the size of the womb is not uniform, for, according to the observations of DESORMEAUX, it is much slower in the earlier months, and much more rapid in the later. According to CAZEAUX, an accurate idea of this increase of the womb may be formed from the following table, which represents the usual dimensions of the womb, at the principal periods of Pregnancy.

	Vertical diameter.	Transverse.	Antero-posterior.
3rd month	$2\frac{3}{4}$ inches	$2\frac{3}{4}$ inches	$2\frac{3}{4}$ inches.
4th "	$3\frac{3}{4}$ "	$3\frac{3}{4}$ "	$3\frac{3}{4}$ "
6th "	$8\frac{3}{4}$ "	$6\frac{1}{4}$ "	$6\frac{1}{4}$ "
9th "	$12\frac{1}{2}$ to $14\frac{1}{2}$ "	$9\frac{1}{2}$ "	$8\frac{3}{4}$ to $9\frac{1}{4}$ "

During the first three months, the womb, from its increase or weight, settles or sinks lower down into the body; its base or upper part is tilted a little backwards, and its neck is advanced slightly forwards; besides, the presence of the large bowel (rectum) on the left side, generally obliges the body of the womb to lean over towards the right, and its neck is consequently directed a little to the left. About the 3d month and a half, or the 4th month, the womb, no longer finding sufficient room below, begins to rise or grow upwards; in doing this, it leans towards the right side, at least 8 times in 10. There are sufficient anatomical reasons for this right lateral obliquity, but most old women think, that the sex of the child exerts a decided influence upon the position of the womb. As the womb rises, the bladder is also gradually pushed upwards, and its neck is more or less compressed, so that an annoying vesical tenesmus is often produced by the pressure exercised upon its neck and body by the womb, the female being tormented by frequent ineffectual efforts to urinate; these demands are always very urgent, and are satisfied with the discharge of a few drops of urine, but are again reproduced, with equal intensity, some minutes after. It is proper to add, that the quantity of the urine is not generally augmented, although some persons, judging from the frequency of the discharges, have thought that it was. It is also right to state, that the irritability of the bladder, in the earliest stages of Pregnancy, proceeds from secondary congestive swelling of the neck of the bladder, rather than from any pressure of the wamb. Pregnant women are also habitually costive, so that a voluminous tumor is apt to be formed by the rectum, when distended with fecal matters, whereby the whole intestinal canal is compressed, and often gives rise to colics, and troubles in digestion. The ovaries, too, being adherent to the womb, are gradually carried upwards, and as they are more sensitive than in the non-pregnant state, and are less protected by the soft walls of the abdomen from external injury, than when low down in the bones of the pelvis, and perhaps also rather more exposed to the influence of cold, we are apt to have attacks of ovarian congestion and inflammation occur, which may be the more readily overlooked and maltreated for colic, as these organs, in the latter months of Pregnancy, are to be found as high up as mid-way between the navel and hip-bones.

As the nerves and sensibilities of the womb are rapidly enlarged and increased during Pregnancy, so are all the distant sensibilities or sympathies of the womb speedily aroused. Amongst these, those of 'the stomach are among the earliest and most common; in fact, nausea and vomiting is so common a symptom, that most females are afflicted with it, and it frequently commences in the very earliest stages; whence many women, taught by their feelings in former Pregnancies, recognize it as an almost certain sign of a new gestation. At times, however, it does not appear till the 3d or 4th month, though seldom later than that; but it is not at all uncommon to see it reappear near the end of Pregnancy, in some who have been frequently tormented in this way, at the beginning.— CAZEAUX.

The breasts, which must be considered as appendages of the uterine organs, quickly commence those changes

PREGNANCY.

preparatory to the accomplishment of the great function to which they are destined soon after delivery; thus, in the very commencement, most women find their breasts to become tender and swell up, and with some, this is so constant a sign, that they do not hesitate to consider themselves *enciente* as soon as it is perceptible. The enlargement is frequently attended by certain pricking sensations or positive pains, sometimes even by engorgement or enlargement of the glands of the arm-pits. About the end of the 2d month, according to MONTGOMERY, but a little later, in the opinion of CAZEAUX. the nipple begins to swell, becoming more erectile, more sensitive, and forms a more marked eminence: its color is also deeper. The surrounding skin becomes the seat of a larger afflux of blood and fluids, it becomes discolored, exhibiting at first a bright yellowish tint, but soon becomes much darker colored. MONTGOMERY, SMELLIE, and HUNTER, thought that the changes which take place in the areola or circle around the nipple, were positive evidences of Pregnancy; and the latter celebrated surgeon, in one extraordinary instance, did not hesitate when examining the dead body of a young female in the dissecting room, to pronounce her pregnant from this sole indication; as the examination proceeded, the hymen was found still intact, but even this had no influence is changing his opinion, and when the womb was opened, its correctness was fully confirmed.—CAZEAUX.

As these changes about the nipple are very important, and easily verified by the woman herself, or at the very least, do not compel a very disagreeable examination on the part of the physician, it is but right to give them in detail. The light, rosy circle around the nipple becomes darker in color, varying in depth of shade according to the complexion of the individual, being generally darker in those who have dark hair and eyes, and in brunettes, than in blonds, or in feeble and delicate women. The circle is from ¾ of an inch, to 1 inch and a quarter in extent; the color grows darker and darker, as Pregnancy advances, and affords anything but an agreeable change to the eye, from the delicately colored areola of the virgin. On the surface of this dark ring, but more especially at that portion of it which surrounds the base of the nipple, a number of small, immature, wart-like elevations, or granules, varying from 12 to 20 in number, soon appear, and attain an elevation of 1 or 2 lines above the surface of the skin. These little knobs are formed by the enlargement of the sebaceous glands about the nipple, and apparently have an excretory duet, because, by pressing upon them, a serous, or serolactescent liquid may be made to ooze out.

At a later period, say about the fifth month, some small, irregularly circular, frekle-like spots begin to show themselves upon the breast, immediately around the dark and warty areola just described, and resembling the stains caused by the sprinkling of a colored liquid, thus constituting another, but spotted and stained areola, which is not so well defined as the first and smaller, darker and granular one, and in fact, it not unfrequently affects a greater part of the skin covering the breast, and then resembles the so-called "moth," or liver spots, which so often appear on the face, neck, and hands of some pregnant women, resembling large freckles. About the same period of time, a number of large veins are seen distributed over the surface of the breast, and send numerous small branches towards the small, dark areola around the nipple, and some of the smaller veins even traverse it. Along the course of these veins, we may *occasionally* observe some brilliant lines, closely resembling those found on the skin of the abdomen of pregnant women, though they are more marked in those females whose breasts were but slightly developed before conception, but had experienced a sudden and rapid increase of size. These silvered threads, or hairs, remain for a longer or shorter period after delivery, and are sometimes serviceable in a medico-legal point of view, in proving that the female has had a child, although they cease to be of any value as a diagnostic sign of her subsequent Pregnancies. These changes about the nipple usually persist during lactation, though when the woman does not suckle her own child, they soon diminish after delivery, but do not wholly disappear; hence they are more conclusive about the first child, than of the others. Whenever they are found, they constitute *an almost certain sign of Pregnancy*, and the physician may pronounce with great confidence the existence of Pregnancy in a young woman who has never borne children, and whose breasts present both a brownish colored areola around the nipple, the granules, or small warts, or tubercles upon this areola, and the freckled appearances around it, just described.—CAZEAUX.

There are also important changes in the *urine* of pregnant women, and probably connected with and dependent upon the changes in the breasts. These changes in the character of the urine are also very important, as they occur at a very early period of Pregnancy, and with a little instruction, may very easily be verified by the woman herself, or if needs be by the physician, without any great encroachment upon the modesty of any sensible married woman. CAZEAUX says: for several years past, the attention of a number of physicians has been directed to certain changes exhibited by the urine of pregnant women, but to NAUCHE is due the principal share of the honor of this discovery; according to this accoucheur:

If the urine of a pregnant woman be received in a wine-glass, and then permitted to settle in a light airy place, a number of little white bodies, or corpuscules, will be found in suspension, but soon subside in the form of cloudy flakes, either on the bottom or sides of the glass, the urine in the meantime becoming more limpid and transparent. This primary deposit does not always occur, and is not absolutely peculiar to the pregnant state; but in the course of 18 of 24 hours, a number of small, brilliant, crystalline granules appear on the surface of the urine; at first, these granules are irregularly isolated, and in some instances unite, so as to form a thin transparent layer, or pellicle, upon the surface of the water, which may only be ovserved when the glass is held obliquely. The urine may remain in this state for several days, though it may soon begin to manifest still more peculiar signs of the presence of Pregnancy. On the 2d, or during the course of the 3d day, the whole of the urine becomes clouded, and a decided scum or pellicle may be discerned, forming at first like a nebulous train, but soon acquiring larger dimensions and greater thickness; all these characteristics are still more evident on the 3d and 4th days, when small particles begin to fall from the scum or pellicle, to the bottom of the glass; by the 5th or 6th day, the first pellicle is almost entirely destroyed, and has settled to the bottom of the vessel, forming a white crust there, but a new pellicle again begins to form on the surface of the urine, less white than the first one, and studded with little brilliant points, having a crystalline lustre, and a greenish tint, in place of the previous milky appearance. In the few succeeding days, the urine evaporates more and more, and becomes thicker and greener; finally, only at this late period putrefaction begins, and the second pellicle is destroyed in turn, to make room for a third, which is not nearly so characteristic in its appearance as the second, and in fact resembles more or less closely that formed on ordinary urine. The characteristic pellicle resembles the layer of fat that floats on the surface of cold broth, and it retains these characters for a long time, and gives off, especially when thick, a strong cheesy odor. The substance forming the pellicle has been denominated *Kiesteine*, (from Χυησις εως, gestation,) by Dr. NAUCHE, signifying the product of Pregnancy; it rarely fails to develope itself in the urine of pregnant women; in 85 cases, it was perfectly distinct in 68; slightly but not very well marked in 11 more; and only absent in 6, in most of whom there were causes sufficient to account for its absence.

The urine of healthy women, who are not pregnant, exhibits nothing similar to this, and if it any time furnishes a pellicle, it has not the distinctive characteristics of Kiesteine. The pellicle, which occasionally forms on the urine of persons affected with consumption, affections of the joints, catarrh of the bladder, or metastatic abcesses, does not appear before the 5th or 6th, and is the product of putrefaction, whereas the true Kiesteine-pellicle appears on the 2d day, is then developed slowly, and is quite independent of putrefaction; its specific gravity is also greater than that produced by any disease whatever. The formation of Kiesteine in the urine is intimately associated with the formation of milk in the breast; Drs. KANE and GOLDING BIRD attribute it to an admixture of milk with the urine, and think that as soon as the least quantity of milk is formed in the breast, it will appear in the urine. Dr. KANE has frequently proved the presence of Kiesteine in the urine, at different periods of Lactation; thus, in 44 suckling women out of 94, the perfect Kiesteinic pellicle was developed, with all the characters it exhibits during Pregnancy, and it was nearly always in those cases where the flow of milk was limited, or rendered difficult by some particular circumstance, and in which the breasts were consequently more or less gorged, that Kiesteine appeared in the urine, but it was found much more rarely after delivery, whenever the mother nursed her infant, or her breasts were properly drawn. In short, the existence of Kiesteine during Pregnancy, and even after delivery, up to the establishment of suckling, and its rare existence during Lactation, and its reappearance when suckling is suspended or impeded, at the time of weaning, for instance, serve to establish an intimate relation between the functions of the breasts, and the Kiesteinic urine.—CAZEAUX. The prevalent theory is, that soon after conception a small quantity of milk is formed in the breast, and as it is not yet wanted for the child, it is absorbed into the system, and thrown out of the body through the agency of the kidneys; in proof of this, it is well known that one of the earliest signs of Pregnancy, is the formation of a small quantity of milk in the breasts, which either oozes from, or may easily be forced from the nipples. TANCHOU has observed Kiesteine in the urine of women who had failed but once in their menstruation; KANE once detected it before the expiration of the 4th week, and again, just prior to the 5th; the peculiar characteristics habitually appear in the second month of Pregnancy, and acquire their greatest development from the 3d to the 6th month. —CAZEAUX.

But the sign upon which most women rely is: *Suppression of the menses.* Most females cease, it is true, to be regular during Pregnancy; and, in fact, this is a law of such general truth, that whenever it occurs in a healthy married woman, without known cause, and is not attended with or followed by disease, it is justly regarded as one of the most certain signs of Pregnancy; but it is not generally known how frequently one profuse menstrual flow occurs soon after conception, and thus obscures the calculation as to the time of delivery. Again, it is not uncommon in some young married women, who had hitherto been quite regular, for the menses to become at once suppressed, and to continue so for several months, without other known cause, than that suppression has probably resulted from the fatigue and excitement of the preparations for marriage, or from the derangement produced by the natural shrinking and fear of modest women, from close contact with man. This accidental and temporary suppression may, or may not, soon be converted into the suppression of Pregnancy; but in both cases, it is frequently accompanied by an augmented volume of the abdomen, together with increased sensitiveness of the breasts, and as the mind so readily believes what it either most ardently desires, or especially dreads, nothing more is wanted in some cases, to found a hope or fear of commencing Pregnancy. Hence the physician must exercise a little discretion, when consulted for an opinion on such a delicate subject. The menses may also continue during the earlier months, or through the whole term of Pregnancy. The subject will be treated of more fully hereafter.

Most women quickly look for some alternation in their size

and shape, as soon as they imagine themselves pregnant; but so many circumstances may cause an augmentation in the size of the abdomen, that but little value can be attached to this sign, unless corroborated by others. In fact, unless there is, as is commonly the case, an increased formation of wind in the stomach and bowels, the lower part of the belly is *flatter* during the first month after conception, than it was before, probably because the womb settles down lower into the hips, from its increased weight. But generally, there is a peculiar, but transient enlargement of the lower part of the abdomen, soon after conception; but this is owing to a collection of wind in the bowels, excited by the neighboring erritation of the womb, and disappears after the lapse of a few weeks, when the bowels have become accustomed to the unwanted stimulus; hence the actually pregnant woman often seems smaller at the end of the 2d month, than during the first. But at the beginning of the 3d month, or at 3 months and a half, the lower part of the body suddenly becomes more prominent, and the enlargement is thenceforth regular and always increasing, up to the full term of gestation.

In the earlier weeks of Pregnancy, the *navel* is also supposed to appear more depressed, or sunken than natural; its base seems to be drawn downwards and backwards, caused probably by the sinking down of the womb into the pelvis, which draws down the top of the bladder with it, and consequently drags upon the urachus, which extends from the bladder to the navel. The circumference of the navel is apt to become the seat of a distressing feeling of weight, and is more sensitive to touch and pressure, and this increased sensibility sometimes extends over a considerable portion of the belly. But at the end of the 3d month, *i.e.*, as soon as the womb begins to rise, the navel resumes its natural condition, and finally becomes decidedly more prominent.

Finally, when Pregnancy occurs, it is generally attended with some slight constitutional disturbance; there is necessarily local congestion, or determination of blood to the womb, for the supprt of the embryo contained within it. The consequence of this increased local action in so important an organ, and one so liberally supplied with blood-vessels, nerves, and absorbents, is, that various symptoms arise affecting the system at large; it is impossible for one part of the system to suffer without some other being almost simultaneously affected. In addition to this local congestion of the womb during Pregnancy, we have for the most part, though not invariably, a state of moderate general plethora: there being, under the circumstances, a greater demand for blood, there is also a tendency to the formation of an increased supply of that important fluid. The whole nervous system is also affected, and in consequence of tnese two causes combined, an irritable (in ordinary healthy cases, we cannot call it febrile) state of the system is induced. The general circulation is more active in pregnant women than in others, and this increased activity manifests itself by a greater frequency of pulse; in fact, it is often harder and more full than in the non-gravid state. The blood drawn from a vein generally exhibits a buffy coat, similar to that in inflammatory diseases, its clot being both more voluminous and more consistent than usual; sometimes, however, it contains a great deal of serum, the clot being small, but still covered with a whitish crust. This condition, which may be considered as the normal one in gestation, is occasionally aggravated, and then general full-bloodedness, or fever may set in.

Pregnancy is also apt to be attended with *changes of moral temperament,* and these changes, for convenience of description, may be divided into, 1st, despondency, 2d, irritability, 3d, hysteria, and 4th, mental derangement.—ANDERSON.

I not unfrequently happens, that women, previously of a happy, cheerful disposition, become low and disponding, and possessed of the most gloomy apprehensions as to the result of their expected delivery. This condition undoubtedly depends upon the peculiar state of the system, existing during Pregnancy, but may be induced in some instances by hearing of, or seeing unfortunate cases occur in friends, or by reading books on midwifery, and fancying that all the worst events therein related must of necessity happen to themselves. Fortunately, this condition often passes off before Parturition occurs.

Sometimes *irritation* of mind predominates, and the patient becomes excited and irritable, and although perfectly conscious of this temporary change in her disposition, has little or no control over its demonstrations; hence every allowance should be made for a misfortune, which is too often considered as *a fault,* and erroneously regarded as perfectly under the control of the patient.

An opposite, and certainly more desirable state occasionally shows itself, for the naturally morose and irritable female may, for a time, assume that mild and happy state, which should be her natural one.

Finally, women who have already had children, have signs, which indicate more or less certainly for them, individually, the commencement of Pregnancy; thus, some always have toothache, styes on the eyelids, or dark spots on the face, neck, and hands, like "moth," or freckles; others are taken at once with salivation, or have strange desires, or longing for unusual articles of food, or sudden fainting fits. HIPPOCRATES thought, that immediately after conception, the eyes become mor sunken and languishing, and surrounded by bluish circles, while the face seemed altered and thinner, and reddish spots, or blotches made their appearance.

The more serious changes of body and mind will be treated of among the disorders of Pregnancy.

MANAGEMENT OF PREGNANCY.

TICKNOR'S rules are:

1. That the woman should avoid all unnecessary, and especially violent exercise, or exertion; such as too fast walking, running, dancing, &c.

2. To avoid all situations which may subject her to unpleasant sights, or seeming dangers.

3. To shun over-heated rooms, and stimulating liquors of every kind.

4. To avoid all substances that have a tendency to produce

a costive state of the bowels, or those which give rise to indigestion, as rich food, late suppers, &c.

5. To take no substances, or drug, that shall give too frequent and too severe motion of the bowels, or such as too severely constipate them, and especially not to disregard the calls of nature, when they may be successfully attended to.

6. To remove from the chest, waist, abdomen, and limbs, every compression or restraint, lest undue pressure should be made upon them.

7. To avoid all substances that may have a tendency to increase the irritability of the system, such as strong tea, coffee, opium, and the too long indulgence in bed.

8. To shun all severe study, and night-watching.

9. To avoid the indulgence of all inordinate appetites.

10. Not to fear that her child will be marked, because certain longings have not been gratified.

11. Not to be apprehensive of evil consequences to her child, because she has been disappointed, or frightened.

12. To guard against any sudden gust of passion.

13. To solicit and attain, as far as possible, tranquility and equanimity of mind.

14. To turn a deaf ear to all tales of disaster, or horror, which purport to have happened to a pregnant womon; for, on investigation, they surely will nearly all prove to be false.

15. Not to indulge in gloomy forebodings, or unreasonable fears for the event; nor to forget how rarely death happens, during, or after a well-conducted labor.

16. Let her make up her mind to bear with manifold inconveniences during her Pregnancy, and some pain at the time of her confinement; and, above all, to feel convinced that the safety of labor does not depend upon the celerity with which it is performed.

17. Let her be passive and obedients, feeling assured that her friends and physician understand and feel for her situation and pains, and will faithfully relieve her of all that can safely be spared her.

18. To examine carefully whether the nipples are of the

proper size and shape; for there is much more danger of suffering with sore nipples, and broken breasts than any more serious affection after confinement. In many instances the nipple is naturally deficient, or has been so thoroughly compressed during girlhood, married life, and Pregnancy, by tight clothing, that after confinement there will be nothing that can properly be called a nipple to be found. The suffering then endured by the mother, if she attempts to nurse her babe, is often dreadfully severe. TRACY suggest a very simple and efficient plan in these cases; it consists in winding a bit of woollen thread or yarn two or three times around the base of the nipple (which has previously been drawn out sufficiently), and tying it moderately tight, but not so tight as to interfere with the free circulation of the blood. Thus, the nipples may be kept permanently and sufficiently prominent; the woollen threads may be worn constantly for many days without the least inconvenience, and with permanent good results.

From the very commencement of Pregnancy a state of mental tranquility is indispensable for the woman. Most women believe that a strong impression upon the mother's mind may communicate itself to the fœtus, producing marks, deformity, &c.; it would be far better for them to believe equally strongly, that anger, jealousy, unfounded repinings and griefs, excessive irritability of mind and temper, &c., may be impressed upon the unborn baby's brain and nervous system, rendering it weakly or nervous, passionate or morose, mischievous or unhappy, &c., &c. It is of the greatest importance that sincere and well-directed efforts should be made, and steadily persevered in, by pregnant females, to keep down those injurious and degrading feelings and irregularities of temper, especially when the exciting causes of them cannot be entirely avoided. Apart from those more serious accidents which are often held up in terror to fractions and obstinate women, the functions of the stomach, liver, &c., are strongly influenced by the mind, and debility, indigestion, jaundice, and various other functional disorders, may be added to the burthen of troubles which almost every pregnant women is called upon to endure as best she may. It is true, indeed, that accidents and misfortunes often bring grief, sorrow, and distress, with a force and pungency that no human heart can altogether resist; but fretfulness and moroseness of temper, envious and jealous feelings, peevishness, hatred, discontent, obstinancy, and perverseness of disposition, are to a certain degree under the control of reason, and a sense of propriety; although every woman and physician knows, that, owing to the unusual irritability of the physical system, induced and maintained by the state of Pregnancy, the difficulty of controlling the feelings often becomes peculiarly great; but, by resisting with constancy and firmness, the indulgence of any thoughts calculated to give rise to any, and all unhappy emotions (for the emotions are in a great measure dependent upon the thoughts), very much may be done to secure both health of body and peace of mind,—TRACY. When the woman has done all that lies in her power, the province of the physician commences. Much may be done by means of remedies addressed to the stomach, liver, bowels, kidneys, or nerves, if these be disordered; still, more may be accomplished by remedies which act directly upon the brain and nervous system.

When there is anxiety, as if from some pending misfortune, Niccol; Kali hyd., Iod., Helleb., Verat, Mezereum, **Anacardium, Clematis, Agaricus, Alumina, Baryta,** or **Arsenicum,** may be indicated.

Those ladies who are exceedingly sensitive about their situation should use Baryta; for, according to Hempel's Complete Repertory, this remedy is indicated when a woman fancies, while walking in the street, that people are laughing at her, and are criticising her, to her disadvantage, so that she dares not look at anybody, and breaks out into a profuse perspiration from shame and fear. This remedy is peculiarly suitable for those mothers who, according to Guernsey, attempt to conceal the rotundity of their form, either from shame or some other reason, with tight dresses, large shawls, or corsets tightly laced.

When there is *anxiety about the future,* CICUTA may be

used, especially if the patient is extremely fearful that something dangerous will occur. If she is exceedingly apprehensive of future suffering, *Laurocerasus* may be given. When there is great anxiety about the future, with sadness and weeping, *Digitalis*. If the patient is apt to become vexed, angry, and impatient, when thinking about the future, *Spigelia*. If she is apprehensive, and thoughtful when thinking about her present state and future destiny, *Anacardium*. When the apprehension amounts to anguish, followed by severe headache, *Æthusa cynapium*.

When *there is a fear of dying*, DIGITALIS and NUX. If she wishes to be alone, and imagines that she will shortly die, *Cuprum*. When she has frequent thoughts of death, *Conium;* with sadness, *Graphite*. When she imagines that she will soon die, although she is not sick, *Nitric acid*. When there is apprehension of death, with difficulty of breathing, *Lobelia*, although Ledum, Rhus, Sulph., Carb. an., Agnus castus, Ammon. c., Ars. Asaf., and Baryta also deserve attention.

When the patient is apt to have strong antipathies against many *persons*, Conium, Cicuta, Aurum, Ammon. mur., and Calcarea may be used. When there is an antipathy against many things, Camphor and Pulsat.

If she is apt to get *angry* at trifles, Bell., Ipec., Cham., Aurum, Nux, Petroleum, and Sepia.

When all her ailments seem very distressing, and she is very dissatisfied, Sepia, Petroleum, Puls., and Aurum.

If she is inclined to find fault with everything, Arsen., Borax, Verat., and China.

If the patient and physician do their part, according to the best of their abilities, the husband must also do his. He must never forget the mutual love which should exist between husband and wife, and that indulgence and charity for all natural defects, tempers, inconveniences, and infirmities of life, with which his wife is now peculiarly beset. No man can form an adequate idea of the manifold inconveniences and annoyances to which a woman is subject while pregnant; and it is incredible how much a wife often has to bear, when she can least endure it, from a husband who is thoughtless, capricious, selfish, haughty, choleric, or dyspeptic, and intractable. Still, however great the trial, the woman should never forget the importance of maintaining a proper state of the mind and feelings; the effects of the contrary course descend to the infant, and often seriously affect, if they do not absolutely determine the general disposition and many of the menal characteristics of the child. Many parents will, unfortunately, have plain and unmistakable illustrations of the truth of this assertion in their own families; it is against the production of mental, rather than physical deformities in their offspring, that pregnant women should be on their guard. The mental state of the mothers of Napoleon and James the First of England, just previous to their confinement, may be cited as apt proofs of the above assumption. Napoleon's mother partook of the dangers of civil war, and is said to have accompanied her husband on horseback on some military expeditions, shortly before being delivered of the future emperor; but the mind of Napoleon's mother appears to have risen in proportion to the danger to which she was exposed, braved it, and triumphed over it; while the circumstances in which Queen Mary was placed were calculated to inspire her with fear alone. The murder of Rizzio was perpetrated by armed men, with many circumstances of violence and terror, in the presence of Mary, Queen of Scotland, shortly before the birth of her son, afterwards James the First, of England; and the constitutional liability of this monarch to emotions of fear, is recorded as a characteristic of his mind; thus, he often started involuntarily at the sight of a drawn sword, while Queen Mary herself was not deficient in courage, and the Stewarts, both before and after James I., were distinguished for their valor, so that his cowardice was an exception to the family character.—RYAN.

Although the popular traditions which render many women exceedingly solici ous test their infants should suffer some *physical deformity*, through the influence of their own minds, has but little truth in it, still it may be expected that

MANAGEMENT OF PREGNANCY. 25

some remarks should be made upon this point. TICKNOR says, it is rather singular that women almost universally believe that a strong impression upon the mother's mind, may communicate itself to the fœtus, producing marks, deformities, &c., while a majority of medical men ridicule the idea as a great absurdity. To set the matter at rest, fairly, the late Dr. WILLIAM HUNTER, of London, investigated this point at the Lying-in Hospital, to which he was attached. In every one of 2000 cases of labor, as soon as the woman was delivered, he inquired of her whether she had been disappointed in any object of her longing, and if she replied in the affirmative, what it was;—whether she had been surprised by any circumstance which had given her an unusual shock, and what that consisted of;—whether she had been alarmed by any object of an unsightly kind, and what that was. Then, after making a note of each of the declarations of the women, either in the affirmative or negative, he carefully examined the child, and affirms, that never in a *single instance* of the 2000, did he meet with a coincidence. He met with blemishes, when no cause was acknowledged, and found none when it had been insisted on.—BULL. But too generally the minds of women are made up upon this subject, and their faith cannot always be shaken by any argument which can be used. The best safeguard against any bad consequences to the mother, is to make a full and candid confession of her fears to her husband, physician, mother, or some judicious friend; but many allow the idea to haunt their imaginations night and day, and become wretched and miserable, because, ashamed of their weakness, they will impart their secret to none; they will hardly confess it to themselves, yet does the impression deepen upon their minds, and they look forward to the period of confinement with the greatest dread and apprehension. Thus, the whole period of Pregnancy is made a season of needless trial, and suffering; and nothing pacifies their minds, or can remove their long-cherished fears, except the birth of an unblemished and healthy child.—BULL. TICKNOR shrewdly advises, if any woman happen to be surprised by an unexpected sight, not to allow her mind to dwell upon it, but to strive to eradicate the impression made, and substitute another in its place; for the power ought to act both ways; so that if it can *mark* it also ought to *unmark*.

TICKNOR also says, that all necessary advice in regard to EXERCISE may be comprised in a few words. Every kind of exercise, or occupation that fatigues, or excites the circulation should be avoided; so also, long walks, lifting, ascending stairs, particularly in a hurry, dancing, riding on horseback, or in a carriage over rough roads. But care must also be taken not to run into the opposite extreme, that of being too inactive. If the custom has been to take considerable exercise before Pregnancy, let it be continued afterwards; only let it be in moderation, such as riding in an easy carriage, walking moderately, and the like. TRACY says, there is an impression in some parts of the country, and more in England than here, that pregnant women should carefully avoid exercise during the *early months,* and take more and more as the time advances. But this is altogether erroneous, for during the first few months, active exercise should be taken daily, to the full extent of the powers of the individual, short, however, of producing such fatigue as to interfere with quiet rest. The exercise taken should be of such a character as will keep the mind intertsted, and the body in more or less constant motion; gentle fatigue should be induced by continued moderate action, and not by violent exertion. Such exercise as this, will operate most favourably as a preventive of a multitude of the bad feelings which are apt to attend this state, and on that account should never be omitted, unless for such reasons as are connected with some peculiarity of the individual; as for instance, a state of disease which renders active exercise impossible without injury to the general health, or a tendency to abortion, when the patient may be obliged to keep very quiet; but even then she should be in the fresh and open air as much as possible. As the time advances beyond the fifth month, the amount of exercise should be diminished, but gradually, until the expiration of the eighth month at least, if not longer; but generally during the last two weeks, the patient feels brighter and easier, and feels more disposition to move about than for some time previously; there are no objections to an increase of exercise then.—TRACY.

Tha DIET should also be well regulated. Notwithstanding the morning sickness and vomiting during the early periods of Pregnancy, the appetite is frequently very craving, especially after the morning sickness has subsided, and an improper indulgence in rich and high-seasoned food, is among the most common errors of females during this period. This error is the more apt to be committed from the incorrect idea entertained by many that, as the child draws its nourishment from the mother's system, a greater quantity of food is required during Pregnancy, than at other times. But there is in many women a strong tendency to a plethoric, or full-blooded state of the system during Pregnancy, which, if not counteracted, either by nausea or vomiting, or a properly regulated and light diet, is very apt to produce unpleasant consequences, such as headache, dizziness, a feeling of fulness, or pressure within the head, and in the veins over the whole system, swelling of the feet and limbs, piles, restlessness, sleepless nights, and numerous other evils arising from the taking of too much, or too nutritious food, and the consequent production of too much blood in the system. These can certainly be no propriety in using such an increased quantity of food that the system becomes oppressed by it. But it sometimes happens that the woman feels best after having eaten more heartily, and then some latitude in diet may be allowed, always doing so with caution, however, and restraining it upon the first occurrence of any of the symptoms of over-feeding.—TRACY. The appetite and taste are generally altered by Pregnancy, and the vulgar attach great importance to the different tastes and longings, and these, as a general rule, may be gratified whenever wholesome aliments are desired. TICKNOR goes even further, and says he has no hesitation in saying, that when the longing is really urgent, the risk of danger from indulging it is much less than it would be from disappointment; provided the craving is not for anything absolutely disgusting, or injurious. It is a fact, though a remarkable one, that, in many cases where the stomach craves really unwholesome articles, they may be taken with impunity. This is well understood by most people; and it is generally believed that ill consequences never result. But this is a great mistake, for TICKNOR has seen the worst effects from this unnatural indulgence; and it must not be forgotten, that when craving for unwholesome articles is to be gratified, it must be done with the greatest caution, and in moderation. When there is an appetite for charcoal, clay, and other articles of this character, the case is one which requires medical advice. A voracious appetite will require a greater quantity of food than ordinary, but never so much as to be injurious; a variable appetite may be satisfied by frequent slight repasts; and a diminished appetite may be stimulated by such food as the woman desires; but it is not necessary for the growth of the fœtus, that the mother should take more food than usual; she may take it to satiety. Every description of high-seasoned food, and the excessive use of wines, liquors, ales, tea, and coffee, are highly injurious, both to the mother and infant. These liquors injure the pregnant woman, and expose her to danger during Parturition, and to fever and inflammation afterwards, while they arrest the growth, and destroy the health of the infant. The simple aliments, of the easiest digestion, and containing the most nutriment in a small volume, are those most appropriate for pregnant women. They should take light repasts, and never overload the stomach. The vulgar prejudice of advising them to take more food than in a state of health, is highly pernicious, and induces indigestion, flatulency, spasms, diarrhœa, and vomiting. As before said, the appetite is capricious, and hence the woman often fancies foods she disliked before conception, and dislikes those she always preferred. Thus, the sight of animal food often disgusts some women for some months. In short, the diet should consist of wholesome articles, such as beef, mutton, lamb, fowl, &c., either roasted

MANAGEMENT OF PREGNANCY.

or boiled, in preference to broiled or baked; and all salted, spiced, or smoked aliment ought to be taken sparingly, or not at all, if the stomach is delicate, as they generally derange it. The flesh of young animals, as veal, lamb, chicken, and certain kinds of fish, are less nutricious than the other articles mentioned, and are therefort considered lighter. Fatty food, as pork, duck, eel, butter, oil, &c., generally disagree with nervous, bilious, or dyspeptic persons, and those who suffer from indigestion, flatulency, and lowness of sprits, and especially during Pregnancy, when there already is more or less tendency to nausea and vomiting. Farinaceous food, such as bread, rice, potato, beans, peas, sago, arrow-root, tapioca, and salep, are highly nutricious, though they may in some cases induce heartburn, flatulency, and indigestion. Mucilagenous aliments, as carrots, turnips, parsnips, cabbages, and asparagus, ought to be taken but sparingly by pregnant women, and those who suckle their infants, and then a little pepper should be used with them. Sweet foods, as sugar, dates fruits, &c., should be used in moderation. Finally, as the stomach is irritable and delicate in most pregnant women during the first months, it is highly necessary, both that their food should be cut small, and then well masticated, to render it more fitted, and more easily acted upon by the stomach; and drink, too, should be used sparingly while eating, for if the gastric juice be too much diluted, it cannot act upon the food in an efficient manner.—RYAN. Most writers, and among them BULL, are very decided about the propriety of moderation in eating; they assume that most persons habitually take more food than is strictly required for the demands of the body, in fact use a superfluity amply sufficient for the wants of the child, for which only a very small quantity is necessary. Nature corroborates this opinion, for almost the first evidence of Pregnancy is the morning sickness, which would seem to declare that only a small quantity of very choice food should be taken. If the appetite in the earlier months in variable and capricious, the woman should not be too readily persuaded to humor and feed its waywardness, for she will very soon bring her system into such a state that it will require a larger supply than is compatible with her own health, and that of her little one. One marked exception may be made to these general rules, viz., when the general health was delicate and feeble before Pregnancy, but becomes invigorated in consequence of this state, and the powers of digestion increase, then a larger supply of nourishment will be demanded and may be met without fear; for instead of being injurious it will be useful. Finally, the female, toward the conclusion of Pregnancy, should be particularly careful not to be persuaded to eat in proportion of two persons, for it may not only bring on vomiting, heartburn, constipation, &c., but will contribute to the difficulties of labor, by the accumulation of impurities in the lower bowels.—BULL.

Some of the alterations in the tastes and appetite of pregnant women require medical treatment. *Cocculus* will be found useful when there is an aversion to food and drink, although the patient is hungry. *Colchicum,* when the repugnance is so great that she shudders eben when looking at food, and still more when smelling it. *Cyclamen,* when food becomes repulsive after swallowing a little of it, followed by nausea. *Gratiola* and *Manganese,* when there is an aversion to food, although it testes well. *China, Arsen,* and *Sepia,* when the thought of food causes nausea. *Sulphur,* when the patient has appetite, but aversion to food sets in on beginning to eat. *Moschus,* when the sight of food makes one sick.

When there is an aversion to *meat,* Alumina, Bellad., Merc., Mezer., and Muriatic acid may prove useful. *Causticum* and *Sulphur,* when fresh meat causes nausea. *Ammon. carb.* and *Zincum,* when there is no desire for meat, or boiled food. *Kali carb.,* when food, especially meat, is repulsive. *Graphite,* when meat and fish are repugnant, although the former tastes well.

We have already alluded to the fastidious tastes, and capricious appetites of pregnant women; some will consider raw oysters a great relish, though, previously to gestation, they could not bear them; others cannot take cheese, although previously fond of it; and some express a vehement desire for fruit out of season, although they never longed for it when it could be procured. One lady always knew when she was with child, by feeling a violent antipathy to wine and tea, which at other times she took with pleasure. Many have a strong aversion to butcher's meat, but one lady has rendered herself celebrated, by a fancy to bite a baker's shoulder, nor could she be satisfied, until the baker's consent was purchased. DEWEES had a patient who was in the constant habit of eating chalk during her whole Pregnancy; her calculation was three half-pecks for each gestation; she finally became nearly as white as the substance itself, and it eventually destroyed her; if she had been well dosed with *Cicuta virosa,* her life might probably have been saved. Another lady took a fancy to gin and water, which she drank in large quantities; her child, when born, was small and lanky, its voice was weak, its face wrinkled and ghastly, and its belly collapsed; its skin was mahogany colored, and hung in folds all over its body; it finally died in convulsions; Arsen., Mosch., Silen., Hepar., or Sepia, might have saved the baby's life, and mother's conscience.

The effects produced on the health of both mother and child, are quite sufficient to show that the mother should come under careful medical treatment, and that, in yielding to these extreme fancies and caprices, we are incurring a mischief, instead of avoiding it. Still the denial should be made with gentleness and moderation, for these caprices generally discover themselves by an air of pensiveness and dejection in the mother; they are often very injurious and absurd, but entirely involuntary, and the woman generally continues anxious and uneasy, till she has obtained her wishes. Frequently, whilst women are under the influence of these desires, all reasoning is thrown away upon them, and, if the proper homœopathic treatment will not remove them, it may be proper to gratify them with the wished-for objects, as abortion has often been the consequence of a disappointment. The success which is said to attend the gratification of their desires, often renders it difficult to deny them, and TULPIUS boastingly cites the case of a woman who devoured 1400 salt herrings during her Pregnancy, and her infant was born equally fond of them, and yet there was not a single mark of a herring, either salt or fresh, upon its body.—CHURCHILL.

In many cases it is evident that the morbid tastes depend upon disorder of the stomach, for the tongue is apt to be coated, or even loaded, the mouth filled with viscid saliva, patient is languid and dejected.

When there is a repugnance to *milk* or *butter*, Carbo veg., Arsen., China, Natrum carb., Puls., Ignatia, Phos., or and there are frequent eructations of glairy fluid, while the Bellad., may prove useful.

When there is an aversion for *sweet things*, Zincum, Sulph., Causticum, and Nitric acid, deserve attention.

When there is aversion to water, Bromine, Tobacco, and China.

Aversion to fish, *Zincum.*

Aversion to vegetables, with desire for meat, Magnesia carb.

Many unnatural desires may be overcome by the aid of medicine. Thus, *Cicuta* is said to remove a great desire to eat coal. *Argen. nit.*, may overcome an urgent desire for strong and acrid cheese. *Sabadilla*, when there is a ravenous desire for sweet things, honey, dishes made of flour, especially when alternating with aversion to meat. *Gratiola*, when the patient relishes bread only. Sabina, Staphysag., Rhus, Chelidonium, Bryon., and Phos. acid, are all said to give a person a great desire and relish for milk. *Hepar. sulph.* may remove a depraved taste for sour, and strong tasting food. *Conium* may be of benefit when the patient only desires coffee, or sour, or salt things. *China, Lycop.*, or *Rhus*, may remove the excessive craving for dainties. Arsen., Mosch., Silenium, Hepar, or Sepia, may aid in removing a depraved taste for brandy, wine, or spirits. Menyanthes and Graphite may help in bring about a healthy appetite for meat. Silex and Verat. may eradicate the craving for raw, cold things, such as cucumbers or pickles, while Opium, Graph., Mosch., or Petrol., may remove an excessive craving for beer, &c.

Dose and Administration.—The same doses and directions, as given for the management of morning sickness, (see page 38), may be followed.

It would seem hardly necessary to make any remarks upon the subject of DRESS during pregnancy; but who has not seen ladies in 'the sixth or seventh month of pregnancy, so tightly laced for the sake of attending a ball or party, as to give but little evidence of their size, or situation; and we must at least enter a protest against this.

It is very important also, to keep the feet and stomach warm, as allowing these parts to be habitually cold, predisposes to colics, abortions, headache, &c.

MORNING SICKNESS.

In the early periods of pregnancy, most women experience more or less of this; and the first intimation of it will most likely be experienced upon rising from bed. Before getting up the patient may feels as well as usual, but while dressing begins to feel nausea, followed by retching, and perhaps by vomiting before leaving the room. Perhaps, it may not occur until some little time after leaving the bed room, or not till after breakfast, which may be eaten with a good relish and almost immediately be thrown up again, with but very little nausea; after which the patient may feel as well as usual until the next morning. This symptom may be present almost immediately after conception, but more frequently it does not commence until after the lapse of two or three weeks, and continues more or less constantly and severely for several weeks, and in some instances, till near the time of quickening, or even until confinement. In some rare instances it does not occur before the last weeks of pregnancy and then is apt to be severe; in other cases it is altogether absent during the whole period of gestation.—TRACY.

In ordinary cases, it is not exceedingly violent and subsides spontaneously about the time of quickening; but sometimes it is excessively severe, continuing for a longer time 'than usual, the irritability of the stomach being excessive; so much so that all food as soon as taken is rejected, and great weakness and emaciation are the result.

Sometimes the vomitings are easy, and without much pain; but at others, they are preceded by such violent and long-continued retchings as to throw the patient into a state of suffering, and extreme agitation; often leaving behind them a distressing pain at the pit of the stomach, which is increased by pressure, and which may at first be mistaken for a symptom of inflammation; but it gradually wears away, and finally disappars sometime after the vomiting has stopped. These shocks and severe strainings are felt at times in the lower portion of the abdomen, and they may give rise to pains in the bowels, or to true uterine contractions, followed by abortion. But in general, such vomitings are only painful and fatiguing to the patient, and should cause no serious alarm. In fact, as CAZEAUX also says that it must not be supposed that these vomitings, even when prolonged, and oft-repeated are necessarily disastrous.

Cause.—The morning-sickness evidently seems due to the sympathetic action of the womb upon the stomach, and does not proceed from derangement of the stomach itself; but when there is undue activity of the liver, there may be more or less bile thrown up with the contents of the stomach. CAZEAUX thinks that in many cases the womb is distended with difficulty, and likewise suffers from this distention, either at the beginning or end of gestation, especially when the enlargement is rendered greater by the presence of twins, or of a large quantity of waters. In the latter stages of pregnancy, it is supposed to be owing to the pressure of the womb upon the stomach. But as the nerves of the womb increase seventy-fold in size from the beginning to the end of pregnancy, the majority of cases are owing to the increased nervous susceptibility of the womb, and the well-known mpathy of the stomach with that organ.

Treatment.—Among the simpler modes of treatment, are: the regulation of the diet, and a change in the times of eating to those hours when the stomach is least apt to be sick. Cold food will sometimes be retained when other kinds are rejected; acid drinks, mineral waters, and swallowing small pieces of ice, have arrested some obstinate cases. CROSERIO recommends

Nux vom. so confidently, that he asserts that a single dose of the 30th dilution in a glass of water, a tea-spoonful, two or three times a day, will ordinarily remove as if by enchantment, all these discomforts, so that the woman will pass through the remaining part of her pregnancy without perceiving them. Still, he gives directions for the use of other remedies in the more severe cases. KROYHER of Presburg, asserts, that what he calls *minute?* doses of Tincture of Nux vomica, are specific against the troublesome vomiting in the early months of pregnancy; in order to ensure success the bowels must be kept gently open, but not purged. He says that Nux will certainly cure the vomiting if it is the sympathetic effect of pregnancy alone; but he advises one or two drops per dose, of the Tincture, gradually increased until ten or more drops are taken every morning in bed, and again in the evening. In many cases it cures in a week, or shorter time; in others it must be used longer. RUECKERT gives five cases cured by Nux; in one case, ½ grain doses of the powder were used; in another, the 3d dilution, and in a third, the 30th dilution.

DEBREYNE thinks the *Colomba* possesses a sort of specific virtue against vomiting, nearly as great as Bark does in agues; but he uses from fifteen to twenty grains per dose, before meals.

TICKNOR recommends *Kreosote,* a few drops in a tumbler full of water, a swallow or two to be taken every half, one, or two hours. WAHLE has cured very obstinate cases with the 6th dilution, with improvement after the second spoonful. CORMACK of Dublin, says it is worthy of notice that Kreosote though excellent in allaying vomiting, often excites nausea and vomiting when they do not exist. Still, he says it is one of the best remedies for stopping vomiting, and seldom fails in the vomiting of pregnancy; he advises from one to three drops, to be taken from five, to ten or fifteen minutes before getting out of bed, and thinks that one dose is often sufficient; but in the more troublesome cases in which nausea and vomiting occur at intervals during the day, a dose should be given every two, three, or four hours. In the vomiting of hysterical persons it is particularly useful; CORMACK used it in ten cases, not only relieving the vomiting, but also calming the general nervous excitement in every case but one.

PULTE recommends *Tabacum,* if with nausea there is fainting and a deadly paleness of the face, relieved by being in the open air; also when the patient loses flesh very fast, and vomits water, or acid liquids, and mucus.

Sepia, if the nausea has lasted a great while, and appears mostly in the morning, and there is a painful feeling of emptiness in the stomach, with burning and stinging. *Sepia* and *Pulsat.* are among the few remedies which act specifically upon both the stomach, and the womb, and hence ought to prove particularly serviceable.

Veratrum was used successfully in four cases; in two cases the 1st dilution was given, in repeated doses.; in one case, the 7th dilution; and in another, the 9th potency. It is recommended when there is excessive sensibility of the nerve of the stomach, and vomiting is excited by the least quantity of water, by moving, or by setting up, and withstands all other remedies; also when the nausea is attended with great thirst, the patient vomiting after drinking ever so little, and having sour eructations, with great debility, and tendency to diarrhœa.

Cuprum and Zinc. when there is little nausea, but severe spasmodic vomiting, and cramps in the stomach or chest set in during the paroxysms of vomiting.

Dose.—1st, 2d, or 3d dilution, every two, four six or eight hours.

Camphor in small doses will often relieve, when a cold perspiration breaks out, the head being hot, and the feet cold.

Dose.—From one to three drops, every one two or four housr.

Secale is recommended when the severity of the vomiting brings on labor-pains, and abortion threatens to set in.

Dose.—From one to three drops of the 1st to the 3d dilution, every five, ten, or fifteen minutes, in severe cases; every one, two, or four hours in milder attacks.

Conium is recommended by CROSERIO when there is decided derangement of the womb; and TROUSSEAU accidentally learned the value of *Belladonna* lotions applied over the region of the womb, in the vomiting of pregnant women, by applying it to a patient who was also suffering with violent uterine pain, with

MORNING SICKNESS.

the effect of relieving both pain and vomiting; in subsequent cases the *Bell.* proved equally serviceable, although no pain was present. They are thought to be particularly serviceable in those cases where there is rigidity of the womb, which dilates and enlarges too slowly for the rapid increase in the size of the child, and thus causes uterine irritation, and sympathetic derangement of the stomach.

Aconite, in drop doses of the Tincture, relieved according to RUECKERT the vomiting of an hysterical pregnant female; she had nausea, retching and vomiting early in the morning; violent colic, and renewed vomiting after every meal, and headache. CHAILLY places great stress upon the presence of inflammation of the decidua, or other uterine membranes, in causing severe and long-continued, and even fatal vomiting in pregnant women. In one of his cases, the patient died in the fourteenth week of pregnancy and had vomited incessantly for three months; the stomach was healthy, but the decidua was evidently inflamed. A second case, also proved fatal in the fourteenth week, vomiting having persisted from the very commencement of pregnancy; there was evident inflammatory engorgement of the decidua and womb, with softening and thickening of the latter. In these cases. *Aconite* may be applied locally over the region of the womb, in the same manner as above recommended for Bellad.; a mere symptomatic treatment of the vomiting will not suffice; the remedies for inflammation of the womb, must also be used.

Ipecac. is recommended by CROSERIO when the vomitings are almost continual, and the woman rejects all, or the greater part of her food, and when she vomits bile, pure or mixed with mucus. He prefers the 6th dilution, repeated three times a day. On two other cases, *Ipec.* 1st dilution was used; and the 2d potency in two more.

DR. ELLIS is in the habit of using Ipec. in doses not to exceed one-eight of a grain, for nausea and vomiting, and rarely fails to quiet the stomach with it.

Aethusa cynapium proved useful in three cases, in which milk could not be borne, but was vomited off, as soon as taken. It was given in the 3d dilution.

Ferrum is thought to be specific when the vomiting occurs after eating, and at no other time.

Dose.—One or two grains of the 1st, 2d, or 3d dilution.

Sulphur was used in four most obstinate and chronic cases, occurring in scrofulous and psoric individuals.

Dose.—The 1st dilution was used in two cases, and repeated six or eight times; the 9th dilution was used in one case.

Hydrocyanic acid is another homœopathic remedy which has become domesticated in allopathic practice; it is supposed to be most indicated when there is great irritability of the stomach, while Nux and Ferrum are conjected to be most suitable, when there is a weak and bloodless state of the stomach owing to the vital energies, nervous and vascular activities being concentrated upon the womb, and hence diverted from the stomach.

Dose and Administration.—The most successful potencies and quantities have already been alluded to in most instances. Of the liquid medicines, such as Nux, Kreosote, Tabacum, Veratrum, Camphor, Secale, Conium, Belladonna, Aconite and Ipecac, from one to five drops of the proper tincture, or dilution may be put in a wine-glass or tumbles half full of water, and from one to three teaspoonsful given every night morning only, when the vomiting and nausea only occur in the morning; and then the morning dose should be given while the patient is still lying down in bed, and as long before rising as convenient. When they occur after every participation in food and drink, a dose should be given from one quarter to half of an hour before each indulgence. When they recur frequently and irregularly at almost any time of the night or day, a dose may be taken whenever the symptoms are most urgent, or after every paroxysm of severe nausea or vomiting.

The dry medicines or powders, such as Sepia, Cuprum, Zincum, Ferrum, and Sulphur may be taken in doses of one or two grains of the proper potency, as often as above directed.

SALIVATION.

This symptom occasionally takes the place of the morning-sickness; it sometimes appears almost at the commencement of pregnancy, and before the time for the expected menses to appear, previous to the fact of their suppression being known;

SALIVATION.

then the woman is apt to feel as if she had taken a slight cold, and as these feelings are often unaccompanied by nausea or any other more common sign of pregnancy, the patient is apt to suppose that her menses have been suppressed by cold. But if she is also troubled with a choking sensation which induces cough, particularly in the morning, and finds her throat and mouth lined with a mucus or saliva of a very peculiar character, she may dismiss the cold-theory from her mind and prepare for something more or less agreeable, as the case may be. This mucus or saliva is very difficult to expel from the mouth; it is extremely white and a little frothy, and when ejected assumes a round shape, about the size of a shilling piece; hence the expression so common in some parts of the country, that "Mrs. So and So, is spitting English shillings, or cotton." When this state of the saliva occurs, it points very certainly to the presence of pregnancy.—TRACY. At other times the salivation is very profuse and severe, so as to resemble the mercurial salivation, but differing from this in the absence of fetor, although the taste may be exceedingly mawkish and disagreeable. It is generally of short duration and disappears of its own accord.

Treatment.—DESORMEAUX says that some candied sugar, or a little gum arabic held constantly in the mouth, will render it less distressing. *Mercurius* is generally regarded as the principal homœopathic remedy.

Dose.—The 1st or 3d dilution may be taken from two to four times a day according to the profusion of the flow of saliva. *Iodine,* is perhaps more homœopathic to this peculiar form of the disorder than Mercury, for the Iodine salivation is without fetor.

Pulsatilla is said to be indicated when it is accompanied with nausea and disgust for food.

Veratrum, when the patient is inclined to be cold and weak, and to be troubled with diarrhœa.

Sulphur will sometimes remove the most obstinata cases.

Digitalis and Nitric acid have also been recommended.

Dose and Administration.—Same as for Mercury. (See above.)

TOOTHACHE.

This may arise from a variety of causes:

1st. And frequently, it and a variety of erratic pains in the face and teeth are induced by the increased irritability of the nervous system, resulting from the new action which is going on in the womb, and in these cases as there is no decay of any particular tooth, the extraction of any tooth for its cure is entirely out of the question.

2d. And also frequently it may arise from decay. A large number of females already have unsound teeth before they become pregnant; and an equally great number are unusually predisposed to rapid caries of the teeth while carrying their children; and in both instances, the above mentioned increased irritability of the nervous system will render them exceedingly subject to frequent and severe attacks of suffering. TRACY says: "There is an impression somewhat prevalent that the extracting of decayed teeth is liable to induce a miscarriage, and it is but just to say that some eminent physicians have this impression." But he is fully satisfied that there is little, if any foundation for it. Excepting in cases where the patient is in very feeble health and her nervous system extremely excitable, he has no more hesitation about extracting them during pregnancy, than at any other time. He believes that in nearly every instance when a miscarriage has followed their extraction, it would have occurred from other causes if the tooth or teeth had not been removed. He has no doubt but that more abortions take place from the irritation caused by decayed teeth, which are allowed to remain for fear of the results of their extraction, than occur from their removal. This is certainly the result of his experience, and some experienced dentists are of the same opinion; they have every year, for many years, extracted a large number of teeth under these circumstances, and so far as they have learned, the operation has resulted unfavourably in no one case. Every danger of abortion may be prevented by the use of a judicious anodyne given one or two hours before the time appointed for the operation.

If the teeth be not too far decayed, the cavities should be cleaned and filled with gold, if possible. In those cases in which the cavity cannot be filled with gold, and it is not advisable to extract the tooth, OSTERMANN's filling may be used—the cavity is to be well cleaned and dried; then forty-eight parts of flocculent Anhydrous phosphoric acid, obtained by bruning Phosphorus under a basin, is to be mixed with fifty-two or fifty-eight parts of pure unslaked lime, and the necessary quantity gently pressed into the tooth. If the tooth be not well dried the mass will become heated, and in expanding will be forced out of its place; and the application must be quickly effected, for the mixture becomes quite hard and useless in the course of two or three minutes. Thus, the cavity will be filled with bone-earth, or Phosphate of lime; and if the filling be be coated over with a few drops of a solution of two drachms of pure Mastich, solved in two drachms of absolute alcohol, and thickened with a proper quantity of powdered silex, a filling will be made which approaches as nearly as possible to the natural structure of the tooth and its enamel.

There are other very good temporary fillings, such as one made by dissolving one scruple of Tannin and five grains of Mastich in two drachms of Ether, then wetting a bit of cotton with it and pressing it into the tooth. Or, powdered West Indian Gum Copal may be dissolved in pure alcohol, by the aid of exposure to moderately warm air, and to this viscid alcoholic solution powdered Asbestos may be added, in place of using cotton. Or, two drachms of picked Mastich, two drachms of absolute alcohol, and nine drachms of dried Balsam of Tolu, may be solved in a stoppered bottle by the aid of great heat, and frequent shaking; when the Balsam is dissolved the whole should be placed in a warm situation, to allow the crude particles to deposite. This mixture is viscid and forms a firm mass, when exposed to the air, which is neither acted upon by the saliva, or other liquids. In order to apply it thoroughly the tooth should be cleansed and dried carefully, and a bit of cotton dropped in the balsam should be put into the cavity; or powdered Asbestos, or powdered Phos. Lime, or powdered Silex may be used in place of the cotton.

If it be absolutely necessary to extract the offending tooth, great care should be exercised in selecting the right one, for the pain sometimes extends sympathetically to a perfectly sound tooth, and is felt but slightly or not at all in the diseased one; and toothache is very often removed by the extraction of a different tooth from the one pointed out as the offending one. TRACY thinks that the diseased tooth will almost invariably be found upon the same side with the painful one, and generally in the same jaw, but not always; an under tooth is often diseased when the pain is seated in a corresponding upper one; and an upper one, when the pain is in the corresponding lower tooth.

3d. The toothache is often secondary to an inflammation of the gum, or:

4th It may be the result of a general catarrhal affection.

The period of the commencement of the toothache, of course varies; certain women suffer with toothache as soon as they have conceived, and even recognize their condition by this symptom; and generally speaking it is a complaint of the earlier months of pregnancy, but some patients have attacks of it throughout the whole period; and sometimes it never occurs until within two or three days of the commencement of labor. The pain varies in degree, and at different times; sometimes it is dull and aching, and ceases at intervals; at others, it is acute and piercing and may continue night and day, so that sleep is lost, the appetite may diminish, the digestion become impaired, the patient become feverish and abortion occur.

Treatment.—This of course will vary according to the nature and seat of the disease. RUECKERT thinks that *Bell.,* Calc., Magnesia and Sepia have proved most useful in the toothache of pregnant women.

ACONITE.

is recommended by KREUSSLER against piercing and throbbing pains in the teeth, when attended with heat and redness of the face, from congestion to the head. Also when the pain is so severe as to drive the patient almost frantic; when the toothache has been excited by exposure to sharp east winds, is attended with fever, quick, hard pulse, mental and bodily restlessness, violent and throbbing pain, generally occupying one side only of the face, but then involving the whole side of one jaw, and attended with redness of the face.—In short, it is a principal remedy in many neuralgic, rheumatic and inflammatory toothaches; I have long been in the habit of applying a small part of a drop of Tinct. of the Root of Aconite, on a bit of cotton to the cavity of aching and decayed teeth, generally with almost immediate relief; I could easily recall a dozen instances in which the pain has been relieved in a very few minutes.

It is often equally successful in purely neuralgic affections of the face and teeth, when the latter are perfectly sound; it must then be applied to the outside of the cheek, or to the gums of the affected part; WATSON speaks very highly of Aconitine ointment in neuralgia of the face; in one case of eight years standing, of very acute neuralgia of the mental branch of the fifth pair of nerves, after exhausting almost every expedient that ever has been recommended for the disease, a permanent cure was effected in six days, by the application of Aconitine ointment, one grain to the drachm of cerate, once or twice a day; in this case no relapse had occurred at the end of six years, although formerly the pain was excited by the slightest causes, such as gentle friction of the hand, or a current of cool air; the patient was soon enabled to face any wind or temperature with impunity.

RUECKERT infers that Aronite is most useful against *throbbing* pains, with congestion to the head, and heat in the face.

Dose.—See treatise on Headaches, page 4; do. on Apoplexy, page 72; Do. on disorders of Menstruations, page 36. In one instance, in a pregnant female, Aconite 200th, quickly relieved a violent and throbbing toothache.

ANTIMONIUM CRUD. ET TARTAR.

MALY found it useful in many intermitting rheumatic toothaches, occurring regular every evening, and not yielding to small doses of Quinine.

Dose.—MALY used one grain doses of the 2d trituration of Antim. Tart., repeated every twelve hours, and always he says with rapid and permanent relief.

ARNICA

of course is used most frequently in pains of the teeth and gums excited by mechanical injuries.

Dose.—One or several drops of the tincture, or of the 1st, 2d, or 3d decimal dilutions may be given every two, four, or six hours.

ARSENICUM,

has a wide-spread reputation against neuralgic and catarrhal toothaches; it is thought to be most useful when the sockets of the teeth are inflamed, the teeth are loose, seem to project from their sockets, and chewing or biting them together produces the sensation as if they were forced into some sore or ulcerated place, the pains being throbbing and piercing, the gums reddened and painful, and all the pains increased by touching, or lying on the painful side, by rest, and cold applications, and relieved by setting up, by restless moving about, and by warm applications; it is still more indicated when the pains quickly produce great debility and exhaustion, the patient being feverish, with coldness of the hands, and especially of the tips of the fingers.

Dose.—The 1st, 2d, or 3d dilution may be given every two, four, six, or eight hours.

AMMON. MURIAT.

WATSON says that this remedy is very useful in a very common very distressing form of face ache, which is sometimes quite intractable under ordinary treatment; it is often called a rheumatic pain, and is probably seated in the periosteum of the jaw, as the extraction of bad or suspected teeth does not remove it; it occupies the lower part of the face, the jaw principally, and the patient cannot say where the pian is most intense. If it does not yield after four doses, no good need be expected from the remedy.

Dose.—WATSON advises half drachm doses, three or four times a day; the 1st, 2d, or 3d dilutions would probably prove equally successful in appropriate cases.

BARYTA.

Was found useful by GASPARY when a pale red swelling of the gum projected into the hollow of decayed teeth, attended with swelling of the cheek, pains extending to the nose, eyes, and temples, and with violent throbbing in the ear.

Dose.—Baryta, c. 8th dilution, one drop per dose, cured a case in four days.

TOOTHACHE.

BELLADONNA.

The indications for the use of this remedy are too well known to require a minute enumeration of them. It is most indicated in feverish, congestive and inflammatory toothaches, both in sound and decayed teeth, when in addition to the excitement of the vascular system there is also great irritability of the nervous system; when there is thirst, dryness and slight redness of the throat and erysipelatous redness of the cheeks; when the pains are much aggravated in the evening and at night, are rending, digging and piercing in their character, and are apt to occur in alternation with intense headache, which almost renders the patient delirious. GARDINER, however thinks Stramonium more useful than Bellad.

Dose.—The 18th or 30th dilutions have been used most frequently.

Hyosciamus is indicatd under nearly similar circumstances.

Dose.—The 9th and 12th dilutions have been given successfully.

BRYONIA.

Many of the indications for the use of this remedy are antagonistic of those pointed out for Arsenicum; thus, Bryonia-pains are increased instead of being relieved by warmth and warm applications, and by lying on the sound side; and they are relieved by cold water, free air, and by lying on the affected side. It is perhaps most useful in rheumatic and catarrhal toothaches, especially when pains in the limbs and chest are also present; when sound teeth are affected in preference to decayed ones, and the pains are apt to shift their locality.

Dose.—The Tincture in solution, the 1st, 3d, 24th and 30th dilutions have all been used with good effect.

CALCAREA CARB.,

Is thought most useful in the tooth-affections of women and children, but especially in those of pregnant females; is serviceable both when the pains are seated in sound or decayed teeth, and when they are exfoliations or growths upon the bone, with more or less disease of the gums. It will relieve, even when there is congestion of blood to the head, and the pains are increased by cold applications, but especially by exposure to a draught of cold air, and when the teeth are unusually sensitive to cold.

Dose.—In one case, a coffee-spoon full of lime water was given several times a day; in 3 cases complicated with fistulous ulceration, the 30th dilution, was given successfully; and in 1 case the 200th potency.

CARBO VEGETABILIS,

Has been used successfully when Merc., and Arsen., seem indicated, but do not effect a perfect cure; especially when the gums become ulcerated, bleed easily, retract from the teeth, and the teeth become loose. Its principal action seems to be directed to the gums.

Dose.—The 9th dilution has been used successfully.

CAUSTICUM.

WEBER says he has cured innumerable cases of toothache with this remedy; it has proved more successful in his hands than any other, even when the pains were felt in all the teeth, or extended over the temples into the forehead. BŒNNINGHAUSEN thinks it most useful against chronic throbbing toothache, when the gums are painful and bleed easily, and the pains extend to the muscles of the face, or to the eye and ear. HERING assumes that it is most serviceable when there is painful looseness and lengthening of the teeth, with fistulæ, suppuration, painful sensitiveness and swelling of the gums.

Dose.—WEBER preferred the 30th dilution; GROSS succeded in one case with the 400th potency.

CHAMOMILLA,

Is an admirable palliative remedy in the most violent attacks of toothache, which seem insupportable and almost drive the patient to desperation; especially if the cheek of the affected side be swollen and red. *Coffea* and *Ignatia* are useful against equally intense pains, without inflammation or swelling, occurring in hysterical women, who are either very quiet, or still and sad. *Dulcamara* is sometimes efficacious against toothache, caused by taking cold and attended with diarrhœa, especially if much saliva collects in the mouth, and Chamomilla seems indicated but does not relieve.

CHINA,

Is said to be the best remedy when toothache is attended with excessive irritability of the whole body, and sleep is disturbed by anxious and frightful dreams; when there is congestion to the head, or excessive paleness and emaciation of the patient, attended with diarrhœa, night-sweat and lassitude.

Dose.—The 1st, 2d or 3d dilution may be given.

COLCHICUM,

Is most useful against rheumatic toothache, when the teeth are sensitive to pressure, and there are rheumatic pains about the jaw and in the maxillary joints, the pains being most severe at night.

Dose.—Same as for Bryonia.

CYCLAMEN.

My friend DR. BELCHER has used this remedy most successfully against pains in decayed teeth, when there is a dull constant ache, with burning in the cheek, followed at times by severe paroxysms of pain, which may drive the patient almost frantic. In some instances the relief was so decided that the patients thought they were more benefitted than they had been by almost any prescription in any other disease. In some cases the relief was very prompt; and in one instance a dull toothache which had lasted a whole night, ceased in a few minutes.

Dose.—The tincture in solution, has been used most frequently.

EUPHORBIUM,

Has been found very useful when the teeth are apt to crumble and break off; also in toothache from decay, when the tooth feels as if it were screwed, or forced into its socket, and is painful to touch, even when gum-boils form, and the cheek is red, swollen and inflamed. Phosphor and Phosphoric acid deserve attention even when the bones of the jaw are involved.

Dose.—The 15th dilution has been used successfully.

FLUORIC ACID,

Has cured fistulæ about the teeth and gums, even when they had lasted as long as three years, and were attended with frequent and violent attacks of pain, with suppuration about the roots of the teeth, with persistent tenderness to pressure.

Dose.—The 3d and 30th dilutions have been used.

KREOSOTE,

Is said to have been used successfully, in the 3d dilution, or even the 24th, when applied to the cavity of decayed teeth, especially when the gums are spongy and ulcerated.

MAGNESIA CARB.,

Has been found very useful by LOBETHAL in those toothaches which occur during the first months of pregnancy; HAHNEMANN also advises it against the toothaches of pregnant women. GUTMANN thinks that it will cure those *chronic* cases in which Chamomilla seems indicated, but fails to afford relief; while RUECKERT thinks it most serviceable against those toothaches in which the pains extend over the whole side of the face, especially when the most violent paroxysms occur at night when the patient is in bed, and force him to rise. It has cured cases which had already lasted for several, or as many as six nights in succession, on the very first day on which it was administered.

Dose.—The 26th and 30th dilutions have been used most frequently.

MERCURIUS.

The indications for the use of this remedy are too well known to require repetition here; suffice it to say that it is not only the most homœpathic remedy against many affections of the teeth and gums, but also has been used more frequently and successfully than any other homœopathic medicine.

Dose.—It has been used in the form of an ointment applied externally; also in the 2d trituration; in the 6th, 9th, 12th and 30th, given in repeated doses; while the 8th and 12th dilution have also been used successfully in solution, in divided doses.

MEZEREUM,

Is most indicated when the periosteum of the sockets of the teeth is most involved, especially when the patient is very apt to feel chilly, and the whole affected side of the head feels cold.

Dose.—The 1st, 12th and 30th dilutions have been used with success.

TOOTHACHE.

NUX VOMICA,

Ignatia, and the North Pole of the Magnet are admirable remedies in nervous and spasmodic toothaches.

Dose.—The 30th dilution has been used successfully in three cases.

PULSATILLA,

Is decided by RUECKERT to be most indicated in the tooth-affections of gentle, quiet, bashful and lachrymose women, especially when the pains are confined to the left side of the face, are of a catarrhal-rheumatic nature, and more apt to attack decayed than sound teeth; also when they extent to the whole of one side of the face, to the ear, neck or head. Pulsatilla-toothaches are apt to be attended with chilliness, paleness of the face, heat, congestion and pain in the head, suppression of the menses, menstrual cramps in the abdomen, anxiety and great restlessness; they are excited or aggravated in the evening or at night, by the warmth of the bed, in a warm room, by warm food, and by sitting or lying down. *Nux-vomica-toothaches* on the contrary are most severe in the morning, are excited or aggravated by exposure to the free cold air, by inhaling cold air, by cold drinks and food, and by mental exertion, and walking about. And vice-versa, Pulsatilla-toothaches are relieved by exposure to the open air, and by holding cold water in the mouth, while Nux-tooth-affections are relieved by warm applications.

Dose.—The 3d, 6th, 7th, 9th, 14th and 15th dilution have all been used successfully.

RHODODENDRON,

Has not been used as frequently as one would suppose from its undouted beneficial effect. It is most beneficial against rheumatic and gouty toothache, when excited by rough, cold and damp weather.

Dose.—In one case the 3d solution relieved in a few hours a toothache which had lasted for fourteen days, in spite of the use of many apparently indicated remedies, in another case it proved equally useful after the pains had persisted for several weeks, with only partial relief from Nux and Merc.

RHUS TOXICODENDRON,

Besides the well known indications for its use, has been found an excellent remedy against caries of the teeth in general, but especially against that form which has received the name of *crusted-caries,* and which is usually connected with herpetic eruptions.

Dose.—The 3d dilution has been used most frequently.

SABINA,

Is homœopathic to the toothaches excited by metastasis of gout from the toes, and also, in those which arise in women who menstruated during pregnancy.

Dose.—The 1st, 2d, or third dilution.

SECALE AND SEPIA

Are suitable against toothaches from sudden suppression of the menses; in chronic throbbing toothaches in women who are annoyed during pregnancy with large yellowish spots over the face, arms and neck; with oppression of the chest, swelling of the face, cough, and enlargement of the glands of the neck. Sepia is also said to be an invaluable remedy against pains in the teeth, in pregnant women, especially when there is great congestion to the head at night.

Dose.—Sepia 30, has been used most frequently.

SILEX,

Has cured enlargement of the bones of the jaw, and inflammation and suppuration about the sockets of the teeth, especially when these parts are more affected than the teeth themselves.

Dose.—Silex 30, has been used most frequently.

SPIGELIA,

Is most indicated against nervous toothaches, especially when burning and rending pains about the zygoma are also present, or pains about the eyes, pressure upon the bladder, palpitation of the heart, and rattling in the chest; or when there are also pains in the eyes and ears, heat in the mouth, and oppression of the stomach.

Dose.—The 3d, 15th, and 30th dilutions have been used successfully.

STAPHYSAGRIA,

Is suitable against caries of the teeth, and inflammations about the periosteum, similar to those in which Cyclamen.

ACIDITY OF THE STOMACH, &c. 51

Mezerium and Rhus, are indicated; but more especially when the teeth become very black, are inclined to crumble off, the gums being white, retracted and swollen, with apthæ, ulcers, and tubercles upon them.

Dose.—The 24th, and 30th dilutions have been given most frequently.

SULPHUR,

Is most indicated against chronic abscesses of the gums, when coupled with considerable growth of proud-flesh, and exuberant granulations.

Dose.—The tincture has been used most frequently; the 30th dilution occasionally.

ACIDITY OF THE STOMACH AND HEARTBURN.

These are very distressing and common symptoms of pregnancy, often occurring very soon after conception; sometimes, however, not until the fourth month; occasionally they are absent altogether, although commonly most troublesome in the latter half of pregnancy.

It is sometimes dependent upon simple irritation of the stomach, attended with a great sense of heat there, at others, by the formation of an acid, which rises into the throat, and from the sensation it causes is called Heartburn. In some cases it is a quite simple affection, and almost every female knows that she may find transient relief by taking a little Magnesia, or chalk, or lime water, with or without milk. But at other times it is a much more complicated affection, which withstands the efforts at relief suggested by ordinary physicians. The acids in the normal gastric juice are:

Muriatic,
Lactic, and
Acetic,—the former predominating, although in varying states of the stomach, either may be in excess and require peculiar treatment. The chyme which is made from the fibrine of meat, and coagulated albumen, contains much muriatic acid; that which is made from quite fresh meat and milk, contains an excess of lactic acid; while that which is made from starch,

farinaceous substances, and vegetables, contains much acetic acid. Hence, some kinds of acidity are aggravated by a meat and milk diet, and relieved by vegetables and fruits, while the more common variety is increased by a vegetable diet.

In some states of the system quite new and unusual acids are formed, or get into the stomach, such as:

Phosphoric acid,
Uric acid,
Oleic, or Butyric acid, and even
Fluoric acid.

The presence of these, of course, calls for quite peculiar treatment. Phosphoric and Uric acids are apt to form in the stomach of those who eat a great deal of meat, and are subject to gout, rheumatism, or nettlerash. Oleic, or Butyric acid is most common in the stomachs of those who indulge in the use of made dishes, hashes, cheese, gravies and fatty food; thus, in the Arctic regions, where the inhabitants live in winter almost exclusively upon seal-fat, fat sea-birds and rancid tallow, a most violent kind of pyrosis, or heartburn, is very common, and doubtless arises from the rancid Butyric acid, which is liberated, or generated in the stomach.

The presence of Fluoric acid is rendered evident by the rapidity with which it attacks the enamel of the teeth, causing caries, especially of the front teeth.

All these different kinds of acids require their specific and peculiar antidotes. The best antidotes for Muriatic acid are Zincum, Ferrum, Argentum and Ammonia, while Soda, Plumbum and Baryta are the best antidotes or Phosphoric acid. The tendency to the formation of Uric acid is best antidoted by Cuprum and Colchicum; while that of Lactic acid is best treated with Zincum.

Again, an *alkaline* stomach is often mistaken for an acid one; for *alkaline dyfspepsia* or pyrosis, as it has frequently been termed, is more common than is generally supposed, at least Dr. Thompson, out of 40 to 50 patients seen daily at the Blenheim Dispensary, generally met with one or two cases per day. There is generally some bilious derangement present, at least the patient is apt to have thirst, or bitter taste in the mouth, as aversion for meat, a craving for sour things, a dirty yellow, or yellowish brown tongue and a dingy sallow skin; it may also be attended with a putrid taste in 'the mouth, eructations like those from spoiled eggs or oysters, and consisting of sulphuretted or phosphoretted hydrogen. In the *acid stomach*, there is said to be a burning sensation at the pit of the stomach, with acid eructations which do *not* alleviate the pain. In the *alkaline stomach*, there is violent pain in that organ, frequently attended with headache and faintness, and a sensation of spasm or constriction of the stomach; this sensation increases until it becomes intolerable, and at last when the agony is complete, the patient is suddenly aroused by a determination to the mouth of a large quantity of fluid, which must be immediately evacuated, to give place to a succession of similar occurrences; at last, however, the flow of fluid becomes so abundant as to constitute an actual stream, and it continues to flow from time to time, but gradually diminishes in quantity, and at length ceases, with complete relief to the pain in the stomach. This relief as characteristic of alkaline indigestion.

Treatment.—PULTE says, that *Nux* and *Pulsatilla* are the principal remedies for dyspepsia, heartburn and acid stomach. For an acid stomach he recommends frequent, but small quantities of Lemonade, or a mixture of one drop of *Sulphuric acid* in a tumbler full of water, and says, that it will sooner and more lastingly correct the acid in the stomach, than lime water or magnesia, which at best only neutralize the acid already in the stomach, without preventing its re-formation. LEADAM recommends Nux 30., three globules to be put in six teaspoonsful of water, and one teaspoonful to be taken three or four times a day, until relieved; but LINNAEUS gave ten drop doses, three times a day with much success. *Pulsatilla* may prove useful when there is an excess, or tendency to an excess of Butyric acid in the stomach. *Sulphur* and *Phosphor* may prove homoeopathic when there is a acidity and flatulence, with an excess of sulphuretted- or phosphoretted hydrogen in the stomach. *Phosphoric acid* has proved more successful than Sulphuric acid is some cases; and a trituration and potency of Gunpowder has often proved more useful than Sulphur, Carbo and Nitrum used singly.

Arsen., Bell., Kali and Calc. have also recommended.

Several Old School physicians have accidentally hit upon the use of *Acids* in heartburn. *Dr. Todd* says, that Heartburn, which is habitual, or of long-standing is sometimes more effectually relieved by *acids*, than alkalies. *Pemberton* mentions having seen it subdued by the juice of half a dozen lemons taken daily, and recurring on the remedy being omitted. *Todd* recommends 5 drop doses of dilute Sulphuric Acid, to be taken every 4 hours; and has also used the dilute Phosphoric Acid successfully. *Billing* says, that alkalies relieve acidity of the stomach for a time but in order to cure it effectually, and *Acid* should be used, such as dilute Sulphuric Acid. *Prout* says, that the injudicious use, and abuse of alkaline remedies, by old school physicians, in acidity of the stomach is often a source of great mischief. Alkalies exert no curative effect; that is, they will not prevent future acidity; on the contrary, when taken in large doses, and at improper times, they cause an absolute increase of acid. Thus, when a large quantity of alkali is taken into an empty stomach, the immediate effect is that this organ in endeavoring to return its natural condition, will throw out an additional quantity of acid in order to neutralize the redundant alkali. When alkaline remedies, therefore, are injudiciously persisted in, a daily contest ensues between the stomach and the self-styled regular doctor. If the constitution be sound, the stomach in spite of the so-called regular doctor, usually gains the ascendancy, but at the expense of extraordinary exertion in the secretion of an excessive quantity of acid. If, on the contrary, the vital process of the stomach be weak, the regular doctor may gain an easy and triumphant victory over the poor stomach, but at the risk of still further enfeebling the vital powers of that organ; an in both instances the general result will be, that the diseased function of the stomach producing acidity will be *augmented*, rather than improved. In Braithwaite's Retrospect, Part 10, we learn that DR. TRACY's experience with the vegetable acids, as corrective of acidity has been considerable; he has prescribed them in a large number of cases, and in nearly all with decided benefit. DR. T. himself was subject to repeated and severe attacks of inflammation of the eyes, accompanied by acidity of the stomach, which he had attempted to correct by the long and free use of Soda, but in vain; it had only a very slight and temporary effect. He had for months abstained from acids, under the impression that they were not suited to his state of health, but was once induced to take a glass of Lemonade, and almost immediately experienced a very copious eructation of gas, with great alleviation. The remedy was again and again repeated with relief to the acidity, and the threatened affections of the eyes were always effectually prevented. TRACY has found the vegetable acids uniformly and entirely successful in removing the disposition to attacks of acidity of the stomach in persons subject to them; and his impression is, that in all such cases they can be relied upon with more confidence than any other remedies. In cases of acidity from pregnancy, he has found sub-acid fruits of great service, while those that are tart could not be borne, and the mineral acids were decidedly injurious, while the whole range of alkalies and absorbents were of little or no avail.

BRAITHWAITE says, this may seem a very unscientific (and equally homœopathic) mode of procedure, but facts seem to corroborate the value of the practice in some cases. DR. CHAPMAN, of Philadelphia, experienced relief from the same treatment, and Professor Wistar informed him, 'that he had for a long time ineffectually endeavored to relieve an opulent merchant, "in the regular way," who was speedily cured by drinking copiously of sour beer, such as had been utterly condemned by the brewers as spoiled and unsaleable. DR. CHAPMAN also had under his care, in consultation, during nearly a whole winter, a most distressing case, which proved utterly intractable to the "regular remedies," which promptly disappeared the next summer as soon as the patient began to subsist upon the sour pie-cherry. Nor is this the only instance in which Dr. C. has heard of cures of acidity of the stomach ascribed to tart, and perhaps unripe fruits of several kinds, and one especially from Professor Hodge, to apples; he also attended a case with DR. RHEA BARTON, which yielded immediately to wheaten mush and vinegar, largely and eagerly consumed.

PAINS AND CRAMPS IN THE STOMACH AND DUODENUM.

UNDER this title BURNS has described an affection not very uncommon with pregnant females; it consists of a cramp-like pain in the region of the stomach and duodenum, occasioning considerable suffering; it may be caused by errors in diet, cold, or by mental emotion, and in some few cases it would appear to be connected with the passage of a gall-stone, and may then give rise to jaundice. Occasionally it is a less simple affection, being complicated with congestion to the head, threatening convulsions, and attended with tenderness of some portion of the spine. (CHURCHILL.)

Pain in the stomach, or Gastrodynia, though generally speaking more transient, is far more severe in its symptoms, and is commonly termed spasm or cramp of the stomach. It is often sudden in its access, and its exciting cause may frequently be traced to some irregularity of diet; the action of cold will also induce it. There are violent neuralgic pains darting through from the breast-bone to the back and shoulders, and not generally confined to the stomach; there is great distension of the stomach and flatulence, and the patient is very restless and anxious. It generally passes off speedily under proper treatment, but occasionally it is somewhat obstinate, and the attacks are particularly apt to be renewed; the soverity of the suffering is so great that it requires speedy and energetic treatment.

CONSTIPATION.

NOTHING is more common, than for pregnancy to change altogether the habit of the bowels; in cases where, previously they were quite regular, or even relaxed, they often become so constipated as to require constant care and attention. The degree, to which the constipation may be carried, varies much; in ordinary cases three or four days intervene between each evacuation; but if the patient be careless about herself, one, two or three weeks, or even months may elapse. This state does not always require that very active treatment, which some physicians consider necessary; the experienced DENMAN says, he was formerly much more assiduous in preventing costiveness than at the present time, having observed, that all women who go on properly, especially in the early part of pregnancy, are liable to this state of the bowels, which may have some relation to the increased action of the womb at that time. Costiveness, may therefore, he assumes, be considered as a state of the bowels corresponding to the increased action of the womb, and will often not prove injurious, as it is a common consequence, and almost necessary result of pregnancy.

Still it is not at all safe to allow it to proceed to the extent which some careless women and prejudiced physicians have fallen into the habit of doing. The most frequent consequences of obstinate constipation are, continued headache, anxiety, giddiness, sleeplessness, distressing dreams, vomiting, displacement of the womb, swellings of the veins of the legs, tedious labor, painful, irregular inefficient pains, obstruction to the passage of the child, and great danger of child-bed fever subsequent to delivery. It also commonly induces general uneasiness, nervous and febrile excitement, loss of appetite, restless nights and erratic pains in the bowels, while abortion may be brought on by the severe efforts and straining required to relieve a loaded bowels of its hardened contents. DENMAN says, that 'there is reason to believe, that this complaint is often overlooked in practice, for it sometimes happens that the mass of indurated and impacted fæces may be enormous, although a small quantity in a liquid state may escape through the free spaces left by them, so that no suspicion of the real state of the case may enter the mind of the woman, or her doctor, unless particular inquiries be made, and the stools be inspected.

By inattention to the state of the bowels some women get themselves into very unpleasant and awkward predicaments; I once attended a newly married lady, who had been over two weeks without any relief from the bowels till finally the rectum and colon became so loaded, that the womb was pushed downwards, and the vagina so much compressed, that the usual social intercourse of married people was entirely out of the question, and both husband and wife came to the conclusion, that some congenital malformation existed. A few does of Castor oil, aided by copious emollient injections soon removed all obstacles. CAPURON met with cases where 'the fæcal matters were so hardened by their long retention in the bowels, that 'they had to be extracted by the fingers and by instruments. CAMPBELL had a case in which the bowels were so overloaded, that after the birth of the child, the attendant thought the woman had another child to bear; the rectum was found distended to the size of a quart bottle, and the woman died of inflammation of the bowels; fourteen pints of fæcal matter were removed after death from the small bowels, after the colon and rectum had been relieved during life. CHURCHILL once attended a labor, in which the hollow of the sacrum was nearly filled up with a hard mass, giving to the finger the sensation of a large growth upon the bone; but a more careful examination proved it to be the lower bowel filled up with hardened fæces; great difficulty was experienced in emptying the bowels, and not until then did labor progress favorably. ASHWELL has known very serious delay during the act of parturition to arise from 'this cause, and has more than once been obliged to empty the rectum mechanically before the head of the child could be propelled into the world.

Hæmorrhoids, or piles are also a frequent consequence of the obstruction offered to the return of blood by this local pressure.

ANDERSON places much stress upon the frequency of occurrence of *rhagades,* or fissures about the anus, combined with spasmodic constriction of the sphincter ani muscle, caused by constipation. Although it occurs in both sexes it is always more common in females than males, owing to the greater neglect with which they treat their bowels, and it is still more common in pregnant females, as constipation is a powerful predisposing cause. It commences insidiously with an irritable itching and burning, and pain confined to one point of the circumference of the anus; the movement of the bowels is attended with excessive pain, which persists for some time afterwards; the sphincter, or closing-muscle of the anus is spasmodically contracted; and the most excruciating pain is experienced on introducing the finger, or a bougie. All these symptoms not only persist obstinately, but increase; the pain becomes more and more severe, lasts longer, and occurs at other times besides during the act of defecation; the contraction of the sphincter becomes more powerful, until finally it is almost impossible to force anything through it; and the patient shrinks from the pain of having her bowels moved; finally, the general health begins to fail, and her life is rendered wretched by such severity of suffering. The fissures are readily discovered on examination.

Causes.—The constipation of pregnant women is generally referred to the effect of the pressure of the enlarged womb upon the bowels; but frequently it is owing to torpor of the bowels, induced by the preponderating current of nervous and vascular energy towards the womb. IMBERT doubts very much whether this compression, which is so much thought about, existing in ordinary cases, for while the womb is seated in the pelvis it is not large enough 'to compress, much less obliterate the rectum ; and when it rises above the cavity of the pelvis, the bowels are behind the womb, and unless the walls of the belly are unusually rigid, they cannot be compressed so as to obliterate their canal. Still, SIEBOLD has mentioned a mode in which the womb exerts pressure on the bowels, which has not been alluded to by other authors, viz., where the vertex, or top of the head of the child, is directed towards one or the other hip, or sacro-iliac synchondrosis, i. e. in the 3th or 4th position of NAEGELE.

Other causes are: the sedentary and indolent habits of many women; cramps of the bowels, arising from increased irritability, and thus retaining the fæces spasmodically; deficiency of bile, caused by frequent and copious vomitings of that fluid.

Treatment.—CROSERIO with characteristic simplicity, thinks that constipation may be generally remedied by a proper diet, by increasing the proportion of vegetables and fruits, or adding the use of a glass of pure fresh water after rising in the morning, and by proper exercise. In those numerous cases in which these means do not suffice, he advises the use of a homœopathic injection of three ounces of water, for the purpose of relieving the rectum of a few small scybalæ, and leaving the rest of the bowels loaded. Still, he and TICKNOR place much stress upon the habit of giving nature a chance to perform her office, by regular attendance every morning at the temple of cloacina, whether 'they experience and urgent call to do so, or not.

When constipation has been allowed to proceed so far as to produce heat in the lower part of the stomach, weight and pressure upon the lower bowel, CROSERIO advises the decidedly inadequate means of giving *Nux vom.* 30th dilution, in the evening, and awaiting its action four or five days; of the effect is not then produced he recommends the use of *Sulphur* 30th, one dose every evening for fifteen days more; and finally in the most rebellious constipation, *Bryonia* 30th dilution, in a glass full of water, a spoonful to be given every two hours, commencing in the morning, until the effect is experienced; in many cases this will probably require fifteen days more. PULTE recommends the alternate use of *Nux, Opium* and *Platina,* one dose of six globules, every three or four hours; until an evacuation is produced; but if many days elapse, or the evacuation be insufficient, he shrewdly observes that a full injection of cold water will probably aid the effect of the medicine. *Bryonia* and *Ignatia* are recommended if the bowels feel painful, and irritation or inflammation is about to set in from procrastinating and insufficient treatment; while *Lycopod.* and *Sulphur* may be tried, if the constipation has already lasted a long time, notwithstanding the above treatment.

Nux-vomica is the remedy most frequently used by homœopathists against constipation, even old school physicians are beginning to use it, claiming it however as an antipathic remedy, on account of its tonic action upon the muscles motor nerves, thus giving tone and vigor to the muscular coat of the stomach and bowels, and necessarily in creating peristaltic action, while it directs again towards the bowels some portion of that nervous energy, which has been drawn in preponderating proportion towards the impregnated womb. BONET says that he has used *Nux-vomica* alone with but slight effect, but has ascertained that an aperient scarcely able by itself to produce a single evacuation, caused active purgation when combined, or alternated with NUX; and thinks that it possesses not only the power of stimulating the muscular fibres of the bowels, but also the property of increasing the activity of medicines that affect the secretions; thus, when added to a single grain of *Mercurius,* it will cause two or three bilious motions; and when combined with a fraction of a grain of Aloes or Rhubarb, it will cause one, or perhaps two full evacuations. He has used *Nux-vomica* as above, for months together and not only experienced no bad consequences, but found the disposition to costiveness materially lessened, while daily relief has been produced during the whole time.

Alumina is another homœopathic remedy against habitual constipation, which old school physicians are beginning to use, ALDRIDGE says it will allay colic, cause alvine evacuations, and promote the secretion of urine, when almost all other remedies fail. PEREIRA says that *Alum* has proved more successful against lead-colic and constipation than any other agent or class of remedies; it allays vomiting, abates flatulence, mitigates pain, opens 'the bowels more certainly than any other remedy, and frequently succeeds in these desirable results, when other powerful drugs have failed.

I have frequently used *Plumbum-aceticum* $\frac{1}{10}$ th, or $\frac{1}{100}$ th with very marked benefit; a dose given once or twice a day for a few days, and then every one, two, four or more days will often overcome the most obstinate and chronic constipation, and the bowels will continue to perform their functions regularly for months without further aid from medicine. But some little adroitness and astuteness is requisite to enable the physician to use this and similar remedies successfully; for constipation may arise from an irritable and spasmodic state of the colon, and a superficial homœopathist may be led to give *Opium*, when he should give *Nux* or *Ignatia;* or it may arise from unusual sluggishness of the muscular coat, or from a sub-paralytic state of the muscular fibres and motar nerves of the bowels, and the routinist will probably give *Nux*, in place of giving *Opium* or *Plumbum*; or it may be caused by, or be connected with a deficient secretion of bile and intestinal fluids, causing a dry state of the bowels, and 'the mere symptomatologist will be as apt to give the antipathic remedies Bryonia, Mercurius and Sulphur, as the homœopathic remedies, Calcarea, Alumina, Plumbum, or Opium.

According to HEMPEL's complete Repertory, *Ferrum-aceticum* is indicated when there is constipation, with piles, and painful pressure while at stool. Ferrum and Plumbum are both homœopathic to constipation from great dryness of 'the bowels, but *Ferrum* is homœopathic to the constipation of ruddy and plethoric persons, while *Plumbum* is homœopathic to that of pale, anæmic, chlorotic, and feeble persons with weak backs, and half paralyzed legs.

Kali bichrom., is indicated in periodical or habitual constipation, when there is pain across the loins, foul tongue, headache and cold extremities.

Capsicum when the constipation proceeds from a heated state of the abdomen.

Moschus is homœopathic to that singular form of constipation which is induced or increased every time one takes Coffee; this article generally exerting or stimulating a laxative effect upon the bowels.

Veratrum, when constipation is caused by an excessive flow of urine, which diverts the fluids from the bowels.

Belladonna, China and *Phosphor* are indicated when there is constipation, with heat is the head, great distension of the abdomen, pressure in the pit of the stomach and dizziness.

Zincum-sulph., has been used very successfclly bp Dr. GEO. STRONG; he gives a does four or five times a day, for one or two days, and then omits the medicine for one or several weeks; three weeks is the shortest period of time within which he has known flatulence and costiveness to return after their disappearance under the use of the *Zinc.* The medicine operates a little singularely; at first there is an increase of flatulence upwoards and downwards, but in a day or two the patiest who may have been so bloated after meals as to be obliged to loosen his waistband, finds himself less bloated, and his wind better for walking, or going up-stairs; soos regular, large, but rarely loose evacuations make their appearance, preceded by a peculiar sensation in the belly, not amounting to griping; occasionally a tingling like the pricking of pains and needles is felt over the body, and even along the limbs, from a vivifying action upon the nerves.

The *Fel-Bovinum-inspissatum* is a most invaluable, natural and non-medicinal palliative remedy against morbid irritability of the stomach, when accompanied by vomiting soon after meals; in acidity of the stomach, with acid and curdled vomitings, gripings and restlessness; and especially against the most obstinate constipation. It prevents milk and other food from turning sour, and immediately dissolves milk again, when it has already coagulated; and is the most rapid solvent of hardened fæces that has yet been discovered; it will soon produce copious motions from the bowels, without the least sickness, or slightest sensation of pain, or even the common feelings of uneasiness or commotion in the bowels. Its efficacy is much increased by giving it in alternation, or combination with Nux-vomca. It is peculiarly serviceable in obstinate constipation of seven, ten or fourteen days' standing; in which a few grains of it will produce

CONSTIPATION.

as much effect as ten or twelve ounces of Castor oil, or from twenty to thirty common purgative pills. Finally, in those very troublesome and serious cases where an immense mass of hardened fæces has become indurated and impacted in the rectum, so that it cannot be moved off by any exertion of the patient, without intense suffering, and which is entirely rebellious to all ordinary injections, so that it generally has been obliged to be dug out with a spoon, a small injection of three or four ounces of ox-gall and water will soon solve and expel the hardened masses pleasantly and effectually.

According to DR. MADDEN (see Brit. Journ. of Hom., Vol. 7, p. 310) the rival systems of Homœopathy and Allopathy stand exactly opposed to each other in the treatment of constipation; thus, while Homœopathy abounds in direct means for ultimately curing constipation, it possesses but few resources for palliation; Allopathy has a countless array of remedies which temporarily remove the difficulty, but scarcely one direct mode of effecting a permanent cure. It is beyond doubt true in the abstract, that laxatives and cathartics ultimately tend to increase the evil which they are given to remove, and that homœopathic remedies which act slowly but directly in restoring natural function, have no such counterbalancing defect. Arguing from these abstract facts, many physicians have uniformly condemned cathartics, and extolled the value of homœopathic remedies; but it not unfrequently happens, that the benefit gained by an immediate unloading of the bowels more than compensates for the subsequent increased tendency to constipation; which in fact may be entirely prevented by using homœopathic remedies in alternation or combination with the aperient MADDEN is convinced, that it not unfrequently happens that a judicious aperient will at once remove a state of things, which if treated otherwise, would entail an illness requiring several days to overcome. There is much unreasonable prejudice among homœopathic practitioners upon this point; they will unhesitatingly condemn the use of the mildest medicinal aperient, and yet will order their patients to eat prunes, figs, roasted apples, green vegetables, brown bread, &c., in hopes of producing the same result. Now, where is the difference? a dose of Castor oil, for example, produces an increased action of the bowels, in virtue of its being an indigestible oil, which passes through the whole intestinal tube almost unchanged, and perhaps exerts a slightly irritating effect upon the mucous membrane, whereas the aliments above named produce the same results in virtue of their having either a large indigestible residuum which irritates by its presence, as is the case with green vegetables and brown bread, or by their containing vegetable acids which directly and specifically irritate the mucous membrane, as is the case with the sub-acid fruits. The result, therefore, is the same in both cases, but in the latter is accompanied with conditions, which render it highly unsuitable in many important cases. It is, however, always objected by the rigid followers of HAHNEMANN, that the one great point to be borne in mind, is that all laxative drugs interfere with the action of our remedies, and hence must be eschewed, however useful they might otherwise be considered; but I (MADDEN) trust, I shall be enabled to prove that both practically and theoreically this interference has been greatly over-rated.

Again, in deciding upon the most suitale treatment for constipation, we must remember that the natural functions of the bowels depend upon various circumstances, all of which must be in operation ere the natural action can be performed. For example, appropriate diet and regular exercise are essential in most instances to produce the desired effect; in spite of this, we often hear of homœopathists refusing any additional aid to patients in whom the confined state of the bowels depends solely upon the absence of these conditions; *e. g.* a person naturally inclined to costiveness, but who by dint of a careful diet and regular exercise has maintained his health, meets with an accident, (breaks his leg, for instance, and hence is confined to bed) and the sudden cessation of his accustomed exercise, checks all tendency to natural action of the bowels, and if frequently happens that the best selected homœopathic remedies will produce no result. What then is to be done? A rigid homœopathist will answer, wait patiently and be guided by the symptoms, and no matter how long time shall elapse without a movement of the bowels, you need not interfere till there is distinct evidence of constipation producing injurious results. In this way, I (MAD. DEN) have heard of six weeks being allowed to elapse without any effort to relieve the patient, and when interference was at

CONSTIPATION.

length imperative, the poor patient had to be delivered of his load, by having it scooped out. Is this justifiable? We may no doubt be told, that cases of nearly as long lasting constipation, have frequently occurred which were not followed by any evil results; but this surely does not warrant our voluntarily permitting a patient to remain in such a condition; for to do this, the advocates of the let-alone system, must be able to prove that it neves does harm, which is quite out of their power. The real question to be answered is this: Do mild aperients do any harm in cases such as above described? all experience proves that they do not, and hence, I, (MADDEN,) believe it to be our duty to resort to them as soon as any necessity for interference exists, provided the homœopathic remedies, fail in producing the desired result. I believe it, as a rule, much safer to secure an action of the bowels, at least every two, three, of four days, even at the expense of administering some mild aperient, than to allow the patient to continue so long in a condition which may at any time become fraught with danger, and which at all times produces much anxiety of mind, in himself and those around him.

There are many other conditions of occasional occurrence, in which homœopathic remedies will fail to relieve constipaton, such as some cases of pregnancy, of congestion of the abdominal veins, of retro-flexion of the womb, and other cases where the cause of the constipation is somewhat mechanical. I, (MADDEN) have met with so many evils resulting from the neglect of the proper regulation of the bowels, by rigid homœopathic practitioners, that I cannot avoid directing very especial attention to this point. About a year ago I was consulted by a lady who had been long an invalid, and had latterly been treated according to our system; her attendant, however, was among the most rigid adherents to all the dogmas of our great master, and accordingly allowed no other means, besides an occasional lavement, to be employed to overcome the great tendency to constipation under which she labored. By degrees the enema lost its effect, and she was then directed to increase the quantity and the frequency of is employment; a number of pelvic symptoms which at this time manifested themselves were attributed by her physician to uterine congestion. When I

(MADDEN) first saw her, she was exceedingly weak, complained of constant drogging pains in the back, which prevented her taking almost any exercise, and the bowels never showed any symptoms of acting, unless she took two or three enemas of a quart each. The lady herself had often thought that the lower bowel was greatly distended; but her physician assured her that her sufferings were uterine; on examination the rectum was enormously distended, extending entirely across 'the posterior wall of the pelvis, and being fully three times its natural diameter. MADDEN.

I, (PETERS) have witnessed several similar cases; one old lady, between 70 and 80 years of age, had been allowed to go several weeks without any movement from the bowels; finally her sufferings became so severe, that she felt compelled to take an anodyne, for which she was severely reprimanded by her strict homœopathic attendant; but many days after she was obliged to resort to the same means in order to obtain a little sleep and cessation of suffering, and the physician immediately abandoned her. When I first saw her she had fever, dryness of the tongue and mouth, great tenderness of the abdomen to touch, and almost agonizing pains in the bowels, most severe at night; the abdomen was so much distended, hard and knotted, that my first impression was, that she had a number of hard malignant tumors of the liver, and mesentery; but equal quantitles of Aloes and Hyosciamus, aided by laxative injections, brought away almost fabulous quantities of fæces, followed by complete relief and rapid recovery, so that I was only obliged to visit her three times in consultation.

DIARRHŒA.

THIS often depends simply upon the nervous irritation induced by pregnancy; at other times it may arise from cold, to which pregnant females are very subject, owing to defect of dress; or from disease of the mucous membrane of the bowels. It sometimes follows conception so closely, that the patient has her attention first drawn by it to her situation, and it may return regularly every month, as though it were vicarious of the menses. CHURCHILL gives the case of a lady who was always seized immediately after conception by diarrhœa, which returned with unfailing regularity every month during the

DIARRHŒA.

whole of her pregnancy, and was often accompanied on its return by violent pains in the stomach. The occurrence of this periodical diarrhœa, was always considered by the lady herself as an indubitable sign of pregnancy; it continued for seven or eight days each month, and on each day she had from fourteen to twenty-five copious discharge, and yet enjoyed a moderately good state of health and spirits. Although we have seen that constipation is most common during pregnancy, yet examples of diarrhœa are very numerous; in fact, however, many of these attacks are caused by previous constipation, and alternate with it; or both diarrhœa and constipation may coexist, for we occasionally find fluid stools discharged while hard fæcal matter is accumulating largely in the bowels. ANDERSON places great stress upon this point, and emphatically urges, that it must not be forgotten that diarrhœa frequently depends upon the presence of extreme constipation; the bowels having been neglected, their mucous membrane becomes irritated by the hardened fæces, over which the watery discharge passes, the indurated masses being unable to come away on account of their size and solidity. In such cases it becomes necessary to break down the scybala by means of injections, or still more mechanical means, such as a spoon, gouge or other instrument.

In the severe cases in which there are inflammation and ulceration of the mucous membrane, the pain is great, often with a sense of internal burning, the pulse is quickened, the tongue dry, skin hot, with much thirst, the oppetite is diminished, and vomiting occasionally occurs; these cases are apt to prove fatal, or cause abortion, about the third month.

PULSATILLA,

Is recommended, if the stools are slimy, greenish and watery, preceded by colicky pains, the mouth being clammy and bitter, without thirst, especially if the patient has chills, and the evacautions occur principally at night.

Dose.—The 12th dilution has been used most frequently, according to Rueckert.

SECALE,

Is also suitable against diarrhœa, when connected with derangement of the uterine organs and suppression of the menses, especially when the passages are slimy and mucous, and the patient's tongue is coated with mucus, with a pasty taste in the mouth, and much rumbling in the bowels.

Dose.—The tincture in water; the 1st trituration; and the 3d and 30th dilutions have all been used successfully.

PHOSPHORUS, AND PHOSPHORIC ACID

Are still more important remedies, when the diarrhœa of pregnant females proves obstinate and chronic, when the passages are painless and half liquid, occasioning general nervous weakness, with some or great emaciation, and progressive undermining of the health.

Dose.—Phosphor. 30 was used successfully in four cases; the tincure in several. Phosphoric acid undiluted, in large and frequent doses, and the 1st to the 9th dilutions have effected cures.

DULCAMARA,

Is indicated when the diarrhœa is caused by taking cold, the passages being greenish or yellowish in color, more or less mucous and acid, being preceded by colic and followed by debility, and generally taking place in the evening.

Dose.—The extract, tincture, 1st, 21st and 30th dilutions have been used successfully.

BRYONIA,

Is recommended when the evacuations are almost involuntary, have a fetid smell and brown color, with much flatulence, especially if caused by taking cold and attended with cough, pain in the side, or rheumatic pains in various parts of the body.

Dose.—The 5th dilution has been used most frequently.

RHUS;

When the passages only occur after midnight.

Dose.—The 1st and other dilutions.

CHINA,

Has proved useful when the passages contain undigested food, and take place soon after a meal, or at night.

Dose.—The tincture, and 12th dilution have been given with success.

ARSENICUM AND SULPHUR

Are often useful in intractable and chronic cases.

Dose.—Ars. has been given in doses of $\frac{1}{80}$ th of a grain; and in the 6th, and 30th dilutions.

JAUNDICE AND LIVER SPOTS.

SOME females acquire a dark, almost yellow color of skin during pregnancy, which must be carefully distinguished from jaundice. Others are often subject to yellow or dingy stains, which occur in patches over the face, or on the forehead, or cheeks.

Treatment.—Sepia, Sulphur, Lycopodium, Phosphor and Arsenicum are the principal remedies.

True jaundice may occur either in the early, or in the later months of pregnancy; in the former case it is probably owing to that sympathy which all the digestive organs have with the impregnated womb; or it may be connected with congestive enlargement of the liver, which continues during pregnancy and terminates with it; or it may arise from inflammation of the liver, occurring accidentally, from cold or mental emotions, such as chagrin.

Symptoms.—In most cases it will be found that the patient has been suffering from a disordered state of the stomach and bowels previously; it often happens that irritation or inflammation of the pyloric orifice of the stomach, and of the duodenum is propagated along the biliary ducts to the liver, and then jaundice is apt to set in after a fit of vomiting, accompanied with tension and weight about the pit of the stomach and region of the liver;—the dyspeptic symptoms are apt to increase after the appearance of the jaundice. In many of these cases the liver will be found enlarged and projecting for one or several inches below the edge of the ribs.

When inflammation of the liver is present, there will be shiverings and flushings, cough, loss of appetite, pain in the right side, with quickness of the pulse, high colored urine and torpid bowels.

When jaundice occurs during the latter months of pregnancy it generally arises from the pressure of the enlarged womb upon the gall duct.

Treatment.—The more simple forms are easily removd by few doses of Mercurius and Chamomilla, in alternation, every two, four, six or eight hours; more obstinate and torpid cases require Sulphur and Nux in alternation every night and morning.

When there is irritation and inflammation of the duodenum, Colchicum is the most homœopathic remedy. When there is congestive enlargement of the liver, Mercurius, Sabina and Aloes are the principal remedies; when the liver is decidedly enlarged, the physician may be rendered anxious about the case, but it is well known, that jaundice and decided enlargement of the liver will often subside spontaneously a few days after delivery. When there is well marked inflammation of the liver, the region of that organ may be freely bathed with the tincture of the root of Aconite, every two, four or six hours according to the severity of the pain, fever and other symptoms, while Aconite, Bellad. and Mercurius should be used internally; in chronic and obstinate inflammation of the liver, Phosphorus is the most homœopathic remedy, although Sulphur and Cuprum may be required in alternation.

HÆMORRHOIDS, OR PILES.

FEW women bear children without becoming in some degree affected with piles. *External* piles rarely given rise to bleeding to any great extent, while *internal* piles are very apt to bleed profusely. Both varieties are apt to become inflamed, and the inflammation may go on to suppuration; when the matter is discharged the abscess may close, and the pile or dilated vein may become obliterated; occasionally the opening remains fistulous, or ulceration of the inner surface of the pile may occur, attended with rather severe and burning pain, lasting for an hour or two after a movement of the bowels, and the sitting posture is often very painful; but the suffering is not nearly so great as that occasioned by an irritable ulcer of the rectum. The patient is also apt to suffer severely at times from the protrusion of the piles, not only after stool, but in a lax state of the sphincters the piles may come down, even when the patient stands or walks about, so as to prove exceedingly troublesome, and interfere with walking exercise. The irritation of piles frequently extends to the urinary organs, the patient being occasionally troubled with a frequent desire to pass water, and even with difficulty in voiding it, from spasm of the membranous portion of the urethra. Although piles in pregnant females are generally caused or aggravated by the pressure of the enlarged womb upon the vessels of the lower bowel, still many females frequently suffer no great inconvenience from them, until irritated by an unusually costive motion, or by the occurrence of an acrid-diarrhœa, or from feverish excitement, when the pile becomes congested and inflamed, and then they have what is termed "an attack of the piles,"—that is to say, they suddenly experience a sensation of heat, weight and fulness just within the rectum, followed by considerable pain at stool, and sometimes by irritation about the bladder. These symptoms, which are often attended with fever, arise from inflammation and swelling of the piles.

When internal piles of some size protrude, they are liable to be constricted and strangulated by the external sphincter; the contracted muscle impedes the return of blood, and occasions inflammatory swelling of the piles, until at length they become strangulated and mortify; an occurrence of this kind is attended with a good deal of pain and suffering, but is generally free from danger.

One of the most common symptoms of *internal* piles is the bleeding, which occurs when the bowels are evacuated. The bleeding varies greatly in amount; sometimes there are only a few drops of blood; in other instances several ounces may be voided. The bleeding may also be irregular, occurring only after costive motions, or in certain states of the health; or it may take place daily, producing the usual symptoms of derangement from continued losses of blood; the complexion may become blanched, and the lips appear waxy; the patient may lose flesh and strength, have a quick and small pulse, suffer from throbbing in the temples, palpitations and difficulty of breathing on making the slightest exertion, and at length finds her legs and feet swollen from œdema. The bleeding may be venous, or arterial in characters; it often unloads the congested and inflamed vessels, and affords the patient much relief; but the bleeding which most commonly occurs from *internal* piles is undoubtedly arterial, taking place from arteries enlarged by the disease. An artery of some side in the sub-mucous tissue may be exposed by ulceration, and continue for some time to pour out blood weakening the patient, and giving rise to the symptoms above described. On examination the surgeon may discover a red, fungous looking mass, from which the bleeding is seen to proceed, and sometimts a small artery may be observed pumping out blood; the blood then has a bright red color, and it is quite a mistaken notion, that bleeding of this character is good for the health of the patient.—(CURLING).

Attacks of piles are most common about the middle, and end of pregnancy, but they may occur at any period. Some women are severely attacked with them immediately after delivery, owing probably to the pressure on, and forcing-down of the bowel during labor.

Treatment.—In cases of internal piles, half a pint of cold water thrown into the bowel in the morning, after breakfact, has a very beneficial effect on the piles by constringing the blood vessels, and softening the motions before the usual evacuations. CURLING says, that the relief afforded by this simple treatment, combined with care in the living, is often remarkable; persons who have suffered more or less from piles years have assured him, that they have been quite free from all annoyance since they have regularly used the cold water lavement. Those who suffer with severe pain for one or several hours after each movement of the bowels, should either lie down for some time after stool, or else change their habit of evacuation to the night, just before bed time, so that they may have entire rest in the recumbent posture.

In many cases there is a slimy discharge and an evidently unhealthy state of the mucous surface of the piles; *Pulsatilla* may be given when there are discharges of blood and mucus, with pains in the back, tendency to diarrhœa and difficulty of urination. *Capsicum,* when there is great irritability of the gastric and intestinal mucous membrane, with burning heat and itching at the anus, with pain and heat during urination. *Copaiba* and *Cubebs,* when there is a profuse discharge of pus, or mucopus from the bowel. Although *Capsicum,* or *red-pepper* is most relied upon by homœopathists, yet in the old school the confection of *black pepper,* better known as *Ward's paste,* has long been in great repute as a remedy for piles, and CURLING says, there can be no doubt, that it exerts a beneficial influence upon the complaint; this preparation is supposed to pass through the alimentary canal but little altered, and on reaching the rectum

HÆMORRHOIDS, OR PILES.

to act directly upon the piles as a stimulating application; the *Cubebs pepper* taken internally seems to relieve piles much in the same way as the confection of black pepper.—(CURLING). In cases where there is much irritation about the mucous membrane of the rectum, great relief may be obtained from the *Balsam of Copaiba*.

When there is much inflammatory irritation with or without discharge of blood, *Aconite* is the most appropriate remedy. *Belladonna* and *Stramonium* are regarded as peculiarly suited for females, when there is hæmorrhoidal constipation from congestion, swelling, or inflammatory irritation of the piles, attended with violen pains in the small of the back, discharge of blood for several days, urgent tenesmus and spasmodic contraction of the anus, with constant pressure and bearing down of the bowel.

Nux and *Ignatia* are most homœopathic when there is much spasmodic irritation of the lower bowel; they are admirable palliatives, when there is a lax state of the sphincters, allowing the piles to protrude when the patient stands or walks. *Ignatia* is most indicated, when the stools are soft; *Nux*, when they are hard and constipated; while *Sulphur* is the most important remedy where there is alternate constipation and diarrhœa.

When there is profuse bleeding from the piles, Sabina, Millefolium and Aloes are the most important remedies.

When there is ulceration of the rectum, *Arsenicum*, *Acid-nitric* and *Acid-muriat*, are the most useful remedies.

In the majority of cases, the alternation of *Nux* and *Sulphur*, one dose every evening, will soon produce a most marked alleviation of all hæmorrhoidal sufferings; if the constipation be very obstinate, *Ignatia* and Opium should be given in alternation every two or three hours until relief is obtained. But I regard *Aloes* as by far the most homœopathic and useful remedy; it may be given in alternation with *Ferrum*, if the loss of blood has already been very great, and a certain amount of Anæmia has been produced. TILT says, that he has never seen piles produced by the frequent use of *Aloes*, but has often seen them relieved by it, and his experience is corroborated by that of GIACOMINI, AVICENNA, STAHL and CULLEN.

Sulphur and *Aloes* in alternation are almost specific against piles, when attended with marked bilious derangement, or torpor of the liver.

Calcarea and *Sulphur* have been given successfully against the consequences of suppression of piles, such as continual vertigo, even when so severe, that the patient is apt to fall down unconscious; congestion of blood to the head, constant aching in the back of the head, palpitation of the heart, great excitabiliy of the whole vascular system, pulsations throughout the whole body, violent, oppressive, stupefying headache, and weakness of memory, with anguish and oppression of the chest from slight physical exertions or moral emotions.

Doses.—Nux has been used successfully in repeated doses of the tincture; also in the 3d and 30th dilutions. *Sulphur* has been most useful when given in the tincture, or 1st trituration, or in doses of $\frac{1}{20}$ of a grain. *Muriatic acid,* in the 1st dilution; *Nitric acid,* in the 5th potency; *Arsenicum,* in the 30th dilution; *Aconite* and *Belladonna* in the tincture, or 1st, 3d dilution.

INCONTINENCE OF URINE.

This inconvenience has already been alluded to, (see page 10). During the early months of pregnancy it generally arises from irritability of the neck of the bladder, or of the entire organ, in consequence of its sympathy with the womb. The patient is tormented with a constant and painful desire to make water; and often, if this desire be not instantly gratified, it is discharged involuntarily. The irritation is sometimes extended to the vulva, and is greatly aggravated by the passage of the urine; the patient may suffer intensely, especially in the night, from scalding, itching and pain of the external genital parts.

It may also arise from pressure of the womb upon the neck of the bladder, giving rise to a partial and temporary paralysis of it. At a later period of gestation, the incontinence is owing to the pressure of the enlarged womb upon the base and body of the bladder, diminishing its capacity, and hence rendering the calls to urinate frequent, be they voluntary or involuntary. This pressure may cause a tedious paralysis of the bladder, so that it may be some time after delivery before its functions are perfectly restored. The incontinence will be much increased, if the patient has a cough, as each paroxysm will be apt to let the urine escape.

In some cases the condition of the patient is very distressing; the constant discharge of urine excoriates the vulva more or less, and the upper part of the thighs, so that the patient cannot move without pain, and the urinous odor may be extremely offensive.

RETENTION OF URINE.

THIS seems to be an opposite condition from incontinence, or inability to retain the urine, yet both are apt to arise from very similar causes. Irritation of the neck of the bladder may give rise to frequent evacuations of urine, or if it proceed to a greater degree, may cause spasmodic constriction, and consequent retention. Pressure upon the neck of the bladder may irritate, or completely compress and obliterate it; pressure upon the body of the bladder may cause paralysis of this, and leave the neck either naturally, or spasmodically contracted. An attack of piles, or swelling of the urethra, may also cause retention of urine.

It is scarcely necessary to describe the symptoms of retention of urine, although a few words may be said about its consequences; these are: difficulty, or inability to evacuate the bladder; great distention of the bladder, so that it presses back upon the womb, and may retrovert, or tilt it backwards; if relief be not afforded, the pain and tension of the bladder may increase to agony, the abdomen become tender, and ultimately the bladder may burst, and the urine be effused into the cavity of the abdomen.

Should retention occur at the commencement of labor, the consequences may be very serious; for the bladder may be forced down into the cavity of the hips by the descent of the child's head, and if it be not ruptured, which is very likely, the bladder will receive such a serious compression and contusion as will doubtless excite inflammation, sloughing and performation subsequently, and all the horrible consequences of vesico-vaginal fistula.

Treatment.—*Nux vomica* is recommended both against retention of urine from paralysis of the bladder, and against incontinence of urine from morbid irritation of the neck of the blodder, with frequent calls to urinate, with pain or urging, without any particular change in the character of the urine. The South Pole of the Magnet has also removed a kind of paralysis of the bladder. *Cicuta,* 3d dilution has cured paralysis of the bladder, with involuntary urination. *Conium* 30, has relieved a painful retention of urine. *Cannabis* has relieved obstinate retention of urine, when accompanied by obstinate constipation.

Cannabis has also relieved the most violent irritation of the bladder, with violent desire to urinate and discharge of a few drops only of bloody and acrid urine. *Cantharides* is homœopathic to a very similar state to the above; also *Capsicum*. *Staphisagria* also relieves painful micturition, when the urine is only passed drop by drop. *Rhus* has cured incontinence of urine, the urine being passed involuntarily unless the desire to pass it is satisfied immediately. *Pulsatilla,* Belllad., Cina, Magnes.-carb. and Antimon.-crud. also deserve attention in obstinate cases. *Dulcamara* is efficient against tenesmus of the bladder brought on, or aggravated by taking cold. *Sulphur* is said to have cured urinary fistula.

SPASM OF THE URETERS.

PREGNANCY females are occasionally subject to accessions of severe-pain in the course of the ureters, leading up to the kidneys, and this CHURCHILL says, DR. BURNS attributes to spasm of the ureters, probably owing to pressure upon these canals as they pass into the cavity of the hips; the attack consists of severe and sometimes intermitting pain, with distressing strangury, which may cause abortion if not relieved. Change of position will sometimes relieve the pain by removing the pressure; if *Cannabis,* Pulsat, or Cantharides do not afford relief, Opium should be resorted to, as it is not only anodyne, but also homœopathic to irritation of the bladder and ureters, and to difficulty or retention of urine. *Camphor* is a useful palliative. These attacks may be mistaken for colic, and for congestion of the ovaries. (See page 10).

ITCHING OF THE VULVA,

is not an uncommon accompaniment of pregnancy, owing probably to the increase of fluids in this part during gestation; at times it is owing to an aphthous or cankered condition of the mucus membrane of the vagina.

Treatment.—Sulphur, Sepia, Opium and Borax are the most important remedies.

ŒDEMA OF THE LABIA,

is rather rare during the early months of pregnancy; it is most common during the seventh, eighth and ninth months. In many cases it is the result of pressure on the veins by the enlarged womb, and is most common in those females who have such large hips that the womb can settle down into the pedvis. In another class of cases it appears as part of a general disposition to dropsy. It is attended with a sensation of fulness, with more or less stiffness of the parts, and difficulty or pain in moving. (See Dropsical affections).

MAURICEAU has described a variety in which there is always considerable itching. Aphthous inflammation may set in, and erysipelas may even occur. Still the whole affection generally disappears soon after delivery.

Treatment.—Arsenicum, Digitalis and Apis-mell. are the most important remedies.

WHITE-WEAKNESS,

or VAGINAL LEUCORRHŒA,

is an extremely frequent accompaniment of pregnancy, so much so, that few females entirely escape, although it is rare for it to produce serious effects. It is worse before the womb rises from the pelvis than subsequently, as it is frequently caused by the gravid womb producing irritation, and by the slow return of the blood from the vagina, owing to the pressure of the womb, coupled with the increased flow of blood to all the sexual parts, which taken place during pregnancy. The state of the patient's constitutional has also much to do with the frequency and severity of leucorrhœa during gestation.

When excessive it causes much debility and aggravates the aching in the back, of which pregnant women so often complain; but at the end of gestation it is said to render the labor more easy, by lubricating and relaxing the passages.

Frequently, the discharge is merely an excess of natural mucus, transparent, colorless and bland; occasionally it is thicker and yellowish and greenish, but rarely acrid; sometimes it is attended with acute inflammation.

Treatment.—*Bovista* is one of the most important remedies; *Sulphur* is said to cure many chronic cases; *Pulsatilla,* when the discharge is thick like cream, and causes itching and irritation; *Sepia,* if the discharge is yellowish, greenish, fetid or corrosive, and attended with bearing-down pains. *Cocculus,* if it is reddish and attended with much colic and flatulency; *Calcarea,* when it is white and corrosive.

DISCHARGE OF WATERY FLUID FROM THE VAGINA.

HYDRORRHŒA, OR FALSE WATERS.

PREGNANT females are occasionally attacked with a fluid discharge from the vagina, quite distinct from the leucorrhœa, which has been described. It may occur, once or several times during pregnancy, and continue for a week or two, or it may persist for several monts.

These discharges are neither preceded or followed by any pains or contractions of the womb; their nature is such as to interfere but slightly with the pregnancy, the latter advancing as usual to its natural term, and at the time of delivery the true bag of waters is regularly formed.

Most generally the female enjoys her usual health before the discharge comes on, when she unexpectedly finds herself wet, the fluid escaping drop by drop, or else she hears the peculiar sound caused by sudden discharge of a considerable quantity of waters. In most eases she suffers no pain either during or after the discharge, though slight uterine contractions may set in; but if the patient keeps perfectly quiet, the pains soon cease and everything resumes its natural order again. The disuharged water are usually a little yellowish, very limpid, and at times tinged with blood, leaving stains upon the linen, and having a well marked spermatic odor. The discharge is much influenced and increased by mental emotions and bodily excitement; on the other hand it augments in quantity during the most perfect quietude, as for instance, at night during sleep. In one case, observed and treated by myself, the discharges only took place at night, during rest or sleep, and then often amounted to one or several pints.

CAZEAUX *supposes,* that the fluid is formed outside of the membranes, between the internal surface of the womb and some portion of the external surface of the membranes, which becomes detached; that is to say, the fluid is secreted from the internal surface of the womb, gradually detaches the membranes, thereby forming a pouch for itself, until its constantly increasing quantity succeeds in separating them as far as the neck of the womb; when a discharge of the fluid takes place. He thinks, that this is the only supposition, which will account for the frequency and abundancy of the discharges, whim rendering the true waters less abundant than usual at the time of confinement, and without there being any marks of laceration of the membranes from careful examination after delivery.

Treatment.—Although this is generally not a serious affection, still it is a very annoying one. CHURCHILL thinks, that nothing can be done except to keep the patient dry, quiet and clean. Arsenicum and Digitalis deserve attention. I once relieved a case with Arsenicum in which there were sudden, frequent and profuse discharges of waters from the vagina.

EXCESS OF WATERS, WITHOUT DISCHARGE.

DROPSY OF THE AMNION.

IN this affection the principal suffering is mechanical, from the pressure of the excessive quantity of Liquor amnii upon the neighbouring parts. The womb is much larger than usual, and proportionably more weighty, rendering the patient very uncomfortable in the upright position and in walking; if the walls of the abdomen be flaccid and weak, the womb may fall forwards, causing what has been called pendulous belly, and adding greatly to the distress. In most cases considerable inconvenience is felt from the increased pressure on the bladder, and upon the stomach and bowels. It would naturally be supposed, that the greater size of the womb and belly would more decidedly obstruct the various veins and blood-vessels of the legs, and cause them and the feet to swell more than usual; but this does not appear to be the case.

The patient's urine is generally scanty; and the infants is very apt to be enfeebled or diseased, or even to die before delivery.

The great distention of the womb sometimes occasions delay in labor, from the too great stretching of the muscular structure of the uterus, and flooding afterwards, from a kind of paralysis from previous over-distention, which interferes with the due contraction of the womb.

Treatment.—The scanty secretion from the kidneys may be increased by the use of Arsenicum, Digitalis, Scillæ, Apis, or Apocynum. (See Dropsical affections).

MENSTRUATION DURING PREGNANCY.

BLOODY discharges are not very uncommon during pregnancy—some females menstruate once of twice after conception in others the discharge returns for four, five or six months, or even during the whole period of gestation. In a few very rare cases the menses appear for the first time during pregnancy, or only during gestation. Churchill thinks that there is not any risk of abortion or premature labor, but these cases should be carefully and anxiously distinguished from those of placental presentation.

CHURCHILL thinks, that they are cases of vicarious menstruation, and that it is neither more or less difficult to account for a monthly discharge of apparently menstrual fluid from the vaginal mucous membrane, than from the mucous membrane of the gums, eyes, ears, or from the surface of an ulcer. (See my Book on Disorders of Menstruation, p. 116). The discharge or secretion may also take place from the internal surface of a portion of the womb, in the same way as suggested, when treating of False waters, or Watery discharges from the Vagina during Pregnancy, see page 78).

WHITEHEAD, however, gives a different and probably very satisfactory explanation; he says, all his patients had leucorrhœa in greater or less degree, accompanied by the train of sympathetic disturbances usua ly attendant upon these affections. This product communicated yellowish stains to the linen upon which it was deposited, and exhibited alkaline properties; evidences of a conclusive character as to its purulent character.

On examination with the speculum, inflammation or ulceration of one or both labia, or of the neck of the womb, complicated in some instances with warty excrescences growing from the neck, or from some part of the viginal membrane, or inflammation of the vagina, &c., was met with in every case, without an exception. Fifteen cases were submitted to vaginal examination while the blood was flowing. In not one of these did any fluid whatever escape from the interior of the womb; the orifice being completely occupied at the time by a plug of transparent mucus. On removing the accumulated secretion by means of a piece of lint, the parts were immediately afterwards covered by a coating of blood, which was distinctly seen issuing from innumerable pores on every part of the diseased surfaces, and soon collected in sufficient quantities to trickle down into the speculum. WHITEHEAD thinks, that his experience is sufficient ly ample to establish as a general rule, that the blood discharged in cases of alleged menstruation during pregnancy is not furnished by the lining membrane of the womb, or by any healthy secreting surface, but by the lower extremity of the womb, external to its cavity, or by the neighboring portions of the vagina, one or the other being in a state of ulceration or suppurative inflammation.

Treatment.—Arsenicum, Cantharides, Argentum-nitricum and Sabina, or Crocus, are the most important remedies, although Cocculus, Kali, Phosphor and Rhus have been used sucessfully. Where there is decided ulceration of the neck of the womb, weak injections of Nitrate of Silver, Bichromate of Potash, Nitrate of Mercury, or of Aurum-, or Stannum-muriaticum may be carefully used.

Mercurius, Nitric-acid, Thuja and Sepia deserve attention, also Kreosote and Sulph.-acid.

UTERINE HÆMORRHAGE.

BLEEDING FROM WOBM.

This is an entirely different and much more serious affection than menstruation during pregnancy. It is almost always either a precursor of abortion, or else is a sign of placental presentation. This can only be decided by carefully watching the case, or by a vaginal examination. In the mean time, the patient should be put to bed immediately, and preserve the horizontal position not only until the complete cessation of the discharge, but until all danger of its return is past. Cold drinks and spare diet should be given: the body kept cool; the covering light, and the room moderate in temperature.

Treatment.—According to Croserio and Leadam, if the bleeding should occur in consequence of a muscular effort to raise or carry anything, a violent exertion of the body, of a misstep, or fall, or blow upon the stomach or back, Arnica should be given, either in the tincture or 3d dilution, and repeated every five, ten or fifteen minutes, according to the urgency of the case.

Ipecac. should be used if the flow of blood is copious, and comes in a continued stream, attended with pains at the navel, bearing down efforts, and pressure upon the womb, and lower bowel, with chills, or general coldness, but heat of the head and face, general lassitude and inclination to lie down.

Dose.—Either sufficient of the tincture or powder should be given produce slight nausea, or else the 3d or 6th dilution may be used every ten or fifteen minutes relief ensues.

Chammomilla may be used, when nearly the same symptoms are present as those mentioned as indicating the use of Ipecac.; especially if the pains are like labor-pains.

Platina, when the blood is black and thick, but not coagulated or grumous; when there is a dragging sensation from the back to the groins, and the internals genitals are exceedingly sore and tender to the touch.

China and *Ferrum* may be given, when the profuseness of the discharge has caused great debility.

Crocus, when the blood is very black, clotted and viscid.

Sabina, when the discharge is bright and red, occurring in jets, followed by the expulsion of clots.

Secale, when he blood is black, tar-like and liquid, and the patient is feeble, and has trembling or cramps of the limbs.

Belladonna, Hyosciamus, or Stramonium, when there is great agitation, excessive vicacity, dimness of vision, some delirium, twitching of the tendons, headache, &c.

N.B. For furher information see my book on *Disorders of Menstruation*, p. 36 to 72, and the Chapter on Abortion in the present work.

RHEUMATISM OF THE WOMB.

THIS may arise from the general causes of rheumatism, such as exposure to cold and wet, inadequate clothing, constitutional tendency, &c.; but besides these, there is a peculiar susceptibility of the wamb to the impression of cold under the attenuated integuments of the abdomen during the latter months of gestation; for the abdomen is only covered at that particular point by very light clothing, and the back, or sacro-lumbar region is often but imperfectly protected by the short jacked, worn by the patient.

Symptoms.—According to CAZEAUX this disease exhibits some well marked peculiarities, by which it can be easily recognied. The principal symptom is pain, or a distressing sensation, which involves the whole, or a part of the womb; its intensity varies from a simple feeling of heaviness to the most painful dragging sensation. When the rheumatism is seated at the top or base of the womb, the pain is particularly apt to be felt about the navel; it is increased by pressure, by the contraction of the walls of the belly, and sometimes even by the weight of the bed clothes; and in many cases the patient is unable to bear any movement whatever. If seated somewhat lower, she suffers from acute dragging sensations that run from the loins towards the lower part of the belly, thighs external genital organs, and the back along the ligaments of the womb. Finally, where the lower portion, or neck of the womb participats in the affection, the seat of it can be detected by vaginal explanation, which, however, given rise to the most acute suffierings. But, of all the causes which may aggravate these pains, there are none more distressing than the incessant movement of the child.

Like all rheumatic pains, those of the womb are wandering, and they occasionally pass rapidly from one of the organ to another; often, indeed, they disappear at once, and pass off to some other part of the body.

They offer frequent and variable exacerbations in their duration and intensity, followed by remissions during which the patient only experiences a vague sensation of heaviness. The womb-pains are usually accompanied by pains in the lower bowel and bladder (recto-vaginal tenesmus), which are the more distressing, the more the rheumatism is located in the lower part of the womb. The patient is then tormented by a continual desire to empty her bladder; the discharge of urine is attended by a smarting sensation, and sometimes by acute suffering, while at others it is even wholly impossible; and in many cases the attempts to move the bowels are equally painful and ineffectual.

The attacks may be attended with chills, fever, extreme agitation and restlessness; towards the end of this paroxysms, a profuse perspiration generally breaks out, which seems to be the prelude of a decided improvement. Then the general and feverish symptoms become moderated together with the pain in the womb; but they reappear with the latter, after a variable period ranging from a few hours to several days.

Influence of Rheumatism of the womb over the progress of Pregnancy.—The paroxysms are apt to be followed by pains and contraction of the womb, and may bring on premature delivery. The patient feels some acute and tensive pains, but this feeling of tension is not uniform; for it increases to an extreme degree, and then becomes weaker. At first the womb becomes hard and contracted, the mouth of the womb may dilate though its dilatation is at first slow and difficult; abortion is then imminent, but it is far from being so frequent as might be supposed; and when it does occur, it is most common when there is decided fever present. The mouth of the womb has been known to dilate to the extent of an inch in liameter, and then the bag of waters, gradually retreated, the womb closed up against, and the abortion did not take place. Consequently, as long as the dilation of the mouth of the womb does not amount to two inches, we may reasonably hope to prevent labor from setting in. These uterine rheumatic pains may simulate those of parturition, and thus lead the practitioner to suspect, that labor has regularly commenced, when in fact such is not the case. The character of the rheumatic pains will aid in preventing such an error. It is probably to some mistakes of this kind, that we must refer those pretended instances of prolonged gestation, as well as those cases, where the genuine travail of parturition was developed, and afterwards suspended during several weeks or months. The influence of this disease over the Labor, and the Puerperal functions will be treated of in a subsequent chapter.

Treatment.—The local application of the tincture of the Root of Aconite over the region of the womb is the most important part of the medical treatment. Aconite may also be used internally, or Bryonia, Pulsatilla, Colchicum, or Mercurius, according to the several and well known indications for the use of these remedies in rheumatic affections.

INFLAMMATION OF THE WOMB.

This is much more frequent during pregnancy than in the unimpregnated state, though less so than after confinement. It very seldom attacks the whole of the womb, except in the early months; the more advanced the pregnancy, the more limited is the affection. It is generally seated in some portion of the body or fundus of the womb, often in that part to which the afterbirth is attached; the muscular tissue is most frequently involved.

Symptoms.—The patient complains of a severe and constant pain or stitch in some part of the enlarged womb, limited generally to a small space; there is tenderness on pressure, increased by walking and by the movements of the child; the pain, unlike that of rheumatism of the womb, does not come on in paroxysms. The bladder and rectum may be sympathetically affected. There is a quick pulse, hot skin, thirst and vomiting.

It may terminate in resolution and the woman go to the full time and be safely delivered; it may terminate in effusion of lymph, firmly uniting the after-birth to the womb, requiring manual assistance to remove it after delivery; it may cause softening of a portion of the womb, followed by rupture during the period of labor; or an abscess may form.—CHURCHILL.

Treatment.—The frequent and free application of the tincture of the Root of Aconite over the region of the inflamel part, is all important.

Nux-vomica has proved a most efficient remedy in HARTMANN's hands, when the fundus, neck, anterior or posterior suface of the womb was the seat of inflammation;—when there was much fever, he gave *Aconite* previous to the use of Nux.

Belladonna and *Mercurius* are also suitable in severe and obstinate cases; while Bryonia and Rhus may be useful, when the serous surfaces are also involved.

Chamomilla and China are useful after the acute symptoms have been subdued, and great nervousness and debility remain.

IRRITABILITY OF THE WOMB.

DEPENDS upon an excited and irritable state of the nerves of the womb, and is nearly allied to hysteria. The symptoms consist of pain in the region of the womb, constant, but occasionally increased in severity, especially after exercise. There is some tenderness to pressure over the pubes, and the womb itself is tender on being touched per vaginam.—ANDERSON.

Treatment.—Agaricus and Stramonium are the most important remedies.

Cicuta-virosa, Cocculus, Conium, Ignatia, Magnesia-muriatica, Nux and Pulsat. are reliable remedies; also Argent.-nit., Bryon, Caust., Cham., Hyosc., Natrum-m., Platina, Sepia and Stannum.

SPASM AND INFLAMMATIONS OF THE WOMB.

THE womb in some cases is affected with pain of a spasmodic character, attended with inflammation; the symptoms are similar to those of irritation of the womb, but far more severe. The pain is evidently spasmodic, and is felt in the back, hips and groins, as well as in the region of the womb; there is great tenderness on pressure, and some fever, and occasionally vomiting.

The result to be feared is abortion, after which in some cases the patient may sink.

Treatment.—Aconite, Belladonna, Stramonium and Secale are the best remedies. Ignatia, Kreosole, Nux-vom. and Thuja also deserve attention.

CRAMPS AND PAINS IN TEH ABDOMEN, BACK, AND LOINS.

PREGNANT women are very subject to pains in the loins—the bearing of the trunk backwards—the efforts made to support the weight of the abdomen, and to maintain the equilibrium of the body, &c. are sufficient to account for these sufferings.

Cramps, spasms, or irregular pains in different parts of the lower half of the body, are a source of frequent and great annoyance to pregnant females. There are various situations in which the cramp or pain is felt, and the effect vary accordingly.

1. *In the abdomen.*—The patient may complain of pain or stitches in one side or the other, generally the left, between the false ribs and the crest of the ilium, or along the lime of the superior insertion of the abdominal muscles. Again, the inferior insertions may be similarily effected; in both cases it appears to be owing to over-distension, which throws some of the muscular fibres into spasmodic action. The pain may be very severe, effectually preventing the patient's taking exercise. It is influenced by the state of the stomach, more than cramp in any other situation, and is often combined with heart-burn or waterbrash; but it is easily listinguished from pain in an internal organ, by its spasmodic character.

CHURCHILL has seen this kind of cramp fix itself about the symphysis pubis, and extend down into the labia pudendi, probably depending upon pressure, congestion, or dragging upon the round ligament.

2. *In the back.*—The lumbar muscles are sometimes the seat

of cramp; and when it is severe, it greatly impedes the movements of the patient, especially the assumption of the upright position.

Occasionally, the distress is extended from the crest of the ilium to the sacrum, affecting the origin of the muscles. It may be the result of distension, or of pressure upon the nerves.

Treatment.—*Nux-vomica* is thought to be generally the best medicine, especially if the severest pains occur just when the patient is going to bed.

Rhus is best suited, when lumbago has been caused by some muscular effort, or by fatigue.

Arnica, when the pains are principally felt when coughing, or walking about.

FALSE PAINS.

SOME women are affected at the latter part of pregnancy with pains somewhat resembling those of parturition, but in reality quite unconnected with it. The causes of these pains are various; they may depend upon flatulence or irritation of the bowels, accompanied either with constipation or diarrhœa, spasm of the bowels, ureters, or biliary ducts, or possibly of the womb itself, and they may be the result of inflammation with accompanying fever. They may be distinguished from true labor pains by their situation and character, the irregularity of their recurrence, and in some instance by their being permanent. On placing the hand over the womb it is not felt growing hard and contracting, as during a true labor pain, and a vaginal examination finds the mouth of the womb closed; or should it by chance be a little open, it does not dilate any more.—ANDERSON.

Treatment.—Pulsatilla, Secale, Balladonna and Stramonium are the most important remedies.

RIGIDITY AND LAXITY OF THE ABDOMEN.

IN first pregnancies we occasionally meet with great rigidity of the abdomen; the womb increases in size, but the abdominal walls do not give way in equal ratio, and a considerable amount of distress is the result. The greatest danger is, that such a degree of pressure will be exerted upon the kidneys as to cause an interfernce with their functions, followed by dropsy and albuminaria.

Laxity of the abdomen generally occurs in women who have borne many children; in these the abdominal walls are so loose, that they are incapable of affording proper support to the enlarged womb, which consequently may fall in any direction.

Treatment.—In *rigidity* of the abdomen frictions with Sweet Oil, or Glycerine, or the application of a Conium-or Belladonna-plaster, coupled with the internal use of Conium, Bellad., or Stramonium will generally suffice.

For laxity of the abdomen, Colocynth and Sepia internally, or dry frictions or frictions with tinsture Nux-vomica, Angustura or Ignatia, together with the internal use of one or the other of these remedies, or of Cuprum and Zincum, Cuprum and Argentum in alternation may prove beneficial.

FALLING OF THE WOMB.

In the early months of pregnancy, when the womb begins to increase in size and weight, falling, or prolapsus is apt to occur; this is attended with a sense of bearing down pain and uneasiness in the lower part of the back, and very frequently in the lower part of the abdomen. This symptom can almost invariably be alleviated and eventually cured by keeping the patient in a recumbent posture. Finally the womb increases so much in size, that it must rise above the brim of the pelvis, there rests, and is of course unable to sink or fall down again during this pregnancy. Sometimes, however, in a more advanced stage of pregnancy, where the hips are unusually large, and the pelvis consequently extremely capacious, a sudden prolapse may occur during some act of unusual exertion.

Both these cases require attention; for in the first the womb having descended, and the patient continuing to go about, it enlarges within the pelvis and gradually becomes impacted therein; —in the 2d instance, the womb becomes at once impacted on account of its larger size.

Treatment.—The bladder must first be emptied by means of

the catheter, and the fallen womb then carefully replaced in its proper situation above the brim of the pelvis; the recumbent position must be persevered in, until the womb is sufficiently enlarged to maintain its location.

Aurum, Bellad., Calc., Kreosot, Merc., Nux-mosch., Nux-vomica, Sepia and Stannum are the principal remedies.

FALLING BACK OF THE WOMB.

RETROVERSION.

The fundus or top of the womb becomes tilted backwards, dropping below the promontory of the sacrum, while the neck of the womb is pushed forwards and upwards, frequently rising above the symphysis pubis, and dragging the vagina up with it. It is most common during the third or fourth month of pregnancy. The rectum or lower bowels is pressed upon by the base of the womb, and the neck of the bladder by the mouth and neck of the uterus; the discharge of urine and fæces being thus interfered with.

Symptoms.—These consist in retention of urine, which frequently sets in somewhat suddenly, and may be either partial or complete. Defecation is performed with difficulty, the fæces being flattened, and coming away in small quantities. When the retention of urine is not complete, only a small quantity is passed at once; there is frequent desire to pass water, but the bladder is never completely emptied; the urine eventually dribbles away involuntarily, and the bladder becomes enormously distended, to a sufficient extent to cause rupture if left to itself; or chronic inflammation of the bladder may set in, even if relieved after the retention has existed for any considerable length of time. There is pain in the small of the back, thighs and pubis, with a sensation of bearing down; and these symptoms coupled with the fact of the patient being in the third or fourth month of pregnancy, should lead one to suspect the nature of the case.

If there be much obstruction of the bladder, fluctuation may be felt above the symphysis pubis. After the bladder has been emptied by the catheter, the womb will not be felt in its natural position in front of the abdomen, above the symphysis pubis.

FALLING BACK OF THE WOMB.

On examination per vaginam, the base of the womb will be felt as a large tumor, lying between the vagina and rectum, and below the promontory of the sacrum; the mouth of the womb can scarcely be reached with the finger, but is found directed upwards and forwards above the symphysis pubis. This, however, is no invariably the case, for the neck of the womb is occasionally very flexible, may be doubled upon itself, and thus leave the mouth in its natural situation while the funds and superior part of the neck are alone retroverted.

A large pelvis, and wide hips may undoubtedly act as predisposing causes to this accident, but they are not by any means essentially necessary; for the womb not having attained a sufficient size in the early months of pregnancy to prevent the possibility of its falling below the promontory of the sacrum, is capable of doing so in a pelvis of ordinary dimensions. A distended bladder may be the immediate cause; this is particularly apt to be the case, whom there is torpor of the bladder, the urine being retained for a long period than natural, and finally voided in large quantities. This torpor is of course a more serious disorder than irritability of this organ, as it is apt to give rise to retroversion. A loaded rectum may also cause tilting back of the womb; sudden contraction of the abdominal muscles, other circumstances being favourable; in fact any thing which can tend to tilt the heavy body and base of the womb backwards, where there is sufficient room for the force of gravity to carry it below the brim of the pelvis.—ANDERSON.

Treatment.—Restoration of the womb to its natural location and direction should be attempted as soon as the nature of the case is made out; the bladder should be emptied at once, and occasionally as soon as this is done, the displaced organ will return spontaneously to its natural position. The rectum should also be thoroughly emptied, and then, if necessary, one or two fingers should be introduced into the rectum and pressed agianst the retroverted fundus of the womb; at the same time, two fingers of the other hand should be introduced into the vagina, and the neck of the womb should be carefully and steadily depressed, while the fundus is elevated. This manipulation may generally be done in the usual obstetric position on the left side; in some rare cases the patient must be placed on her hands and knees,.

in order to get the influence of the force of gravity; in others, the uterine-sound must be used.

Nux, Ignatia, Bellad., and Aurum are all serviceable remedies. The patient should learn to lie upon her face, always at night and frequen'ly during the day time.

ANTIVERSION.

IN this, the body of the womb is thrown forwards; it is exceedingly uncommon during pregnancy. The symptoms are similar to those of retroversion, but the signs on examination are entirely different. The enlarged womb may be felt above the pubis, and the neck of the womb is found directed backwards towards the promontory of the sacrum.

Treatment.—The patient should practice lying upon the back, with the knees drawn up. The bladder and lower bowel should be regularly and methodically emptied. A bandage and compress over the pubes may be serviceable; the funds of the womb may be pressed back, and neck pushed forwards by the physician.

FŒTAL TURBULENCE.

THE motions of the unborn child are generally felt at four months, or four and a half months;* frequently these movements are exceedingly feeble, at first only producing a kind of tickling, or rather a sensation analogous to that which a spider's claws excite in crawling; at other times they are veritable shocks, which may be violent enough to elicit cries from the mother; occasionally they become so violent as to be truly distressing, causing a sense of nausea, often attended with local pain, and much general nervous agitation. ANDERSON thinks that this affection may depend upon some preternatural sensibility of the womb itself, but more frequently it arises from a

* Of seventy cases the motions of the child were felt at the end of the third month in mine cases; at three and a half months in eleven cases; at the fourth month in twenty-one cases; at four and a half months in sixteen cases; not until the fifth month in eight; cases; at five and a half months in one case; in the sixth month in four cases.

state of general nervous irritation, which is from time to time determined to the womb.

Treatment.—Mechanical compression by means of an abdominal bandage will frequently prove of much service. Agaricus or Stramonium may remove the morbid sensibility of the womb; while a general nervous condition may be alleviated by Chamomilla, Sumbul, Cannabis-Indica, Coffea, &c.

PALPITATION OF THE HEART.

CHURCHILL says, that almost all females suffer from attacks of palpitation at some period or other of their pregnancy, especially those of a weakly, delicate body, or nervous temperament. By some it is felt immediately after conception, and some even have attacks after ordinary intercourse; by others it is only felt at the period of quickening; and by a third class towards the end of pregnancy.

Among the exciting causes may be enumerated mental emotions, disordered stomach and bowels, especially errors of diet and flatulency; the motions of the child often give rise to it.

Symptoms.—The attack may come on suddenly, or be preceded by some nervous or gastric disorder; the patient feels the heart strike violently against the ribs, so as to shake the whole body; in general the heart's action is regular, although excessive; but in some cases a marked and frequent intermission may be observed. If asleep when the attack occurs, the starts up suddenly; and if walking is obliged to stand still; the breathing becomes hurried or impeded, the nervous system may be disturbed by headache, giddiness, dimness of vision, noises in the ears, and sensation of approaching apoplexy.—CHURCHILL.

It is not dangerous, although often distressing; for the hard and increased acion the heart may be either very sudden, and violent, or persist night and day, for many days.

Treatment.—As it may be produced by excitement of the mind and derangement of the digestive organs, the diet should be carefully regulated, and the mind kept at rest; some severe attacks only subside after full, free and spontaneous vomiting; if it arises from indigestion accompanied with much flatulence and acidity, almost immediate temporary relief may be obtained by the administration of an alkali. *Sarsaparilla* is useful when there is painful palpitation; *Zincum,* when there is a painful palpitation, with sharp stitches at every beat of the heart; also *Agaricus and Hepar-sulph. Veratrum and Nitric-acid,* when there is diarrhœa, anxiety, and hurried breathing *Aurum* and *Asparagus,* when there is anxiety and oppression of the chest, with lowness of spirits. Nitrate of Silver, when there is palpitation with faintness and nausea. *Ammonia-carb.,* when there is a weak and sinking feeling at the pit of the stomach. *Gratiola,* when there is such violent palpitation, that the whole body is shaken; also *Crocus* and *Secale. Spigelia* and *Sabadilla,* when there is palpitatiin, with throbbing in the abdomen, and over the whole body. *Mercurialis,* when there is an undulating and throbbing motion in the stomach and abdomen, with pulsation of the abdominal aorta, and dizziness.

FAINTING.

Is not a frequent occurence during gestation, except perhaps at the time of quickening, and in the weakly, and delicate. It is ordinarily of no great importance; when organic disease of the heart is present, it is very serious. Towards the end of pregnancy, fainting is regarded with great suspicion, not so much for the immediate consequences, as for its effect upon the convalescence after parturition. It is also a very unpleasant occurrence at the time of labor; it sometimes follows each pain, causing great alarm, but without apparently retarding the progress of delivery; but after delivery, from slight over-exertion, or from too active aperient medicine, fatal fainting may set in.

Ordinary fainting after confinement may easily be distinguished from fainting in consequence of internal hæmorrhage; the latter is more prolonged, accompanied with fulness and tension of the abdomen, dull weight and pain in the pelvic region, permanent blanching of the surface, and after a short time by escape of blood from the vagina.

Treatment.—When there are repeated fainting fits, *Cuprum* and *Hyosciamus.—Arsenicum, Camphor, Ammonia, Cocculus,*

SPITTING OF BLOOD. 95

Moschus, Veratrum, Stramonium, Laurocerasus, Ferrum-acet., Nux, Petroleum and *Opium* all deserve attention.

DIFFICULTY OF BREATHING.

May occur during the early months from a nervous affection and sympathy with the womb; it is also often connected with the nervous palpitations already treated of; the attacks are generally, short, sudden, and not attended with plethora, congestion or fever.

In the middle of pregnancy it is more frequently owing to plethora, and the face is apt to be flushed, the pulse quick, head heavy, &c.

In the latter months it generally arises from the pressure of the enlarging womb; it is then apt to be most severe in first pregnancies, owing to the resistance afforded by the abdomen in expanding for the first time to so great an extent.

The attacks are not serious unless complicated with congestion, inflammation, or organic disease of the lungs.

Treatment.—*Moschus,* Ipecac. and Aconite are the most important remedies.

COUGH.

The cough, which is peculiar to pregnancy only, occurs in the earlier and latter months; it is either constant, short and teasing, or recurs in violent paroxysms, causing great distress and inconvenience.

In the earlier months it is generally nervous, spasmodic and sympathetic; there is rarely any expectoration, and no evidence of catarrh, or disease of the lungs. In the latter months it is owing to a mechanical cause; the aorta is compressed, the circulation through the lungs somewhat arrested, and the lungs irritated and rendered uneasy.

Treatment.—*Conium* is the principal remedy. *Ipecac, Drosera, Ferrum-acet., Pulsatilla, Petroleum,* Plumbum-acet., *Ruta, Mezereum, Cino* and *Sepia all* deserve attention.

SPITTING OF BLOOD.

THIS formidable disorder is fortunately very rare; in the earlier months the attack may be simple, consisting of a secretion of blood from the mucous membrane of the air tubes, owing probably to the sudden suppression of menstruation.

In the middle or latter months it may arise from congestion of the lungs; or more frequenly from consumption, which often runs its course quietly, and unnoticed during pregnancy.

Treatment.—*Aconite, Stibium* and *Ipecac.* are the principal remedies; although *Phosphor, Kreosote, Hamamelis* and *Millefolium* deserve attention. *Mercurius-solubilis, Arnica, Arsenicum, Zincum, Digitalis, Ferrum-aceticum* and *Hepar-sulph.* have been used successfully.

HEADACHE.

CHURCHILL says, that next to disturbance of the stomach, headache is probably the most common complaint of pregnant women. In the early months it is generally of a nervous character; at a later period it must frequently arises from plethora.

In nervous headache there is seldom any quickness of pulse, suffusion of the eye, or flushing of the face; in headache from plethora the pulse is full, quick and strong, the face flushed, the eyes bright or suffused, the eyelids heavy and closed, and there may be intolerance of light and sound. In some congestive headaches, however, the face is pale.

Either variety may arise from constipation; or from scantiness of the urine.

Treatment.—See *Teatise on Headaches. Pulsatilla, Stramonium, Sepia, Aconitum, &.c.* deserve attention.

SLEEPLESSNESS.

CHURCHILL says, there is scarcely a more distressing complaint to which pregnant women are subject, than sleeplessness. It is not uncommon, and appears chiefly to attack females of a delicate constitution, or of a nervous temperament. It may occur at an early period of pregnancy, though it is more common during the latter months, and may persist for a considerable time.

It generally seems to be a purely nervous affection, excited by want of exercise, excessive motion of the child, or uneasy sensation in the womb; sometimes, however, it arises from a plethoric and feverish state of the system.

If it persist long, the patient will suffer severely; become restless, feverish, agitated, peevish and fanciful; her appetite will diminish, the bowels and secretions generally become deranged; the skin get hot and dry, and the pulse quick; she will complain of great weakness and misery, and ultimately her judgment and mental facul.ies will become impaired.

Sometimes the patient will sleep well in the day; but not at night. At other times the rest is disturbed by frightful dreams.

Treatment.—Air and exercise are very important; a draught of cold water just as the patient steps into bed, or wrapping a wet towel around one hand, or bathing the feet at bedtime, will often calm the nervous irritation.

Rhus is the best remedy, when the patient cannot sleep before midnight. *Ranunculus-scel.*, when she always wakes after midnight. *Plumbum,* for obstinate sleeplessness for weeks together. *Moschus,* when there is no sleep all night, or only momentary losses of consciousness. *Mercurius,* when she sleeps much in the daytime, but cannot sleep at night. *Ledum* and Hyosciamus, when sleep is constantly interrupted by starting. *Causticum,* when she wakes every morning at four o'clock. *Aconite,* when there is sleeplessness from pain. *Veratrum.* when there is an intolerable feeling of heat, and restless tossing about. *Ambra* and *Agaricus,* when there is sleeplessness from great activity of mind and nervousness; also *Chammomi la.* *Graphite,* when she cannot sleep before two o'clock at night. *Fluoric-acid,* when there is no sleep until towards morning, and then a very little slumber is sufficient to refresh the patient. *Bryonia* and Causticum, when there is sleeplessness from vascular excitement, and dry heat. *Digitalis,* when there is uneasy sleep, from constant desire to urinate. *Cuprum,* when there is much vomiting. *Laurocerasus,* when there is loss of sleep from excitement and attacks of heat. *Nitric-acid,* when icy coldness of the feet prevent sleep. *Borax,* when sleep is disturbed by thirst and coldness of the body. *Anacardium,* when there are severe pains in the abdomen.

HYPOCHONDRIASIS.

Has been sufficiently treated of at p. 22 & 23

PLETHORA.

Has been alluded to on p. 18. Acute serous plethora is not uncommon during pregnancy, and is apt to be attended with bloating not only of the legs and feet, but also of the face, arms and hands; it then is a most serious disorders, being often complicated with albuminuria and retention of urea in the system, to be followed by severe headache, violent vomiting, and pain at the pit of the stomach, and is too often succeeded by convulsions.

Treatment.—*Aconite, Sulphur, Aurum, Digitalis* anl *Kali-carbonicum.*

DROPSICAL AFFECTIONS.

DROPSY OF THE LEGS.

According to Churchill during the latter months of pregnancy we frequently find patients complaining of a swelling of the feet or legs, increasing towards evening, and occasioning a certain amount of inconvenience. This dropsical swelling may be confined to the feet and legs, or it may involve the thighs, vulva, and hips. In the majority of these cases the swelling is caused by the pressure of the gravid uterus simply. When the effusion is the result of pressure, there are none but mechanical symptoms; the limb is swollen, and of a semi-transparent, pearly appearance; it feels heavy, and the patient cannot walk as well as usual. These inconveniences are much aggravated if the swelling extends to the thighs; the patient may not be able to approximate them, and may find it as distressing to sit, as to stand, or walk. But little additional distress is occasioned during pregnancy by the swelling of the labia; but if very large they may prove a very serious impediment to the exit of the child during labor. Change of posture has a great effect upon the swelling of the legs; in the morning it is but slightly perceptible, but during the day it increases, and towards night it arrives at its maximum. After delivery the effusion disappears quickly; but previously it may be unpleasantly varied by an attack of erysipelas, or phlegmonous inflammation of the cellular tissue.

GENERAL DROPSY OF THE SKIN. (*Anasaraca*).—In a few cases the dropsy is more general and extends to the upper part of the body, and to the hands and face. If the urine be scanty or albuminous the case should be narrowly watched. Albuminuria, or Bright's disease, according to DEVILLIERS and REGNAULT is not a frequent complication of pregnancy, but when it is present, œdema and eclampsia are the most frequent indications of its presence. Albuminuria and its effects are more common in first than in later labors, and then generally disappear after delivery. Dropsy of the face and hands, going on occasionally to general anasarea, is one the most frequent accompaniments of albuminuria in the pregnant female. Albuminuria, when present during the last months of pregnancy, denotes a marked tendency to puerperal convulsions. Every case of puerperal convulsions seen by M. BLOT was accompanied by albuminuria. The Albuminuria of pregnancy is generally attended with dropsy of the face and hands, and lumbar pains; it is almost always unattended by fever; is in most cases the result of a simple functional hyperalmia of the kidneys, and disappears a few hours after delivery; this condition of pregnancy is free from danger as long as it is uncomplicated with congestion of the brain; but if severe headache and a peculiarly severe pain in the pit of the stomach be attended with profuse bilious vomiting in a pregnant female, in the latter months of gestation, albuminous urine also being present, then we may almost certainly expect an attack of puerpual convulsions.

Treatment.—*Arsenicum* is useful against elastic swellings; also when there is swelling of the face and feet, with dryness of the month and lips, distension of the abdomen, diarrhœa, colic and vomiting; or swelling of the right sight of the body down to the hip, with swelling of the left foot and leg; or swelling of the face and body.

China, when there is swelling of the limbs. *Ledum-palustre,* when there is œdematous swelling of the whole body. *Lactuca-virosa,* when there is a dropsical swelling of the whole body, with asthmatic complains, heaviness of the head, difficulty in lying down, chills, shortness of breath, hacking cough and small slow pulse. *Sepia,* in chronic cases, when there is a swelling of the wrist, elbow and ankle joints in the evening; or swelling of the whole body, face, belly, legs and arms, extending down to the wrist-joints, with shortness of breath, fever, and alterations of chills and heat; also when there is swelling of the labia, followed by a moist and itching eruption upon the inner surface. *Digitalis,* when there is an elastic and painful swelling of the legs, followed by a similar state of the arms and forearms, slowly passing off, after some months, without increased secretion of urine; or when there is an elastic, white swelling of the whole body, with painfulness to the touch, followed after many weeks by anasarca, with great softness of the swelling. *Rhus-toxicodendron,* is most homœopathic against acute inflammatory œdema, especially of the face and eyelids; but it has also been used successfully in large doses, against torpid and chronic anasarca. *Apis-mell.,* is indicated under almost similar circumstances to those which call for *Rhus, Mezereum* or *Cantharides.* *Hellebore* is also useful in chronic dropsy. *Secale*-cornut, is homœopathic to watery, soft and painful swellings. *Crotalus* in swelling of the whole body.

HARTMANN regards *Digitalis* and *Scilla* as mere palliatives in dropsy; he thinks, that *Cantharides* may prove useful, when there is much irritation of the bladder; *Kali-carb.* is pronounced indispensable, when Anasarca and Ascites are consequent upon suppression of the menses. *Zincum-metallicum,* when there is great distress in the region of the kidneys. *Colchicum,* when dropsy has been caused by suppressed perspiration, from exposure to cold, damp and foggy weather, or from getting wet through to the skin; *Dulcamara* deserves attention under the same circumstances; and *Colchicum* is peculiarly homœopathic to the severe pain in the stomach and violent bilious vomiting, which is apt to precede an attack of convulsions,

DROPSICAL AFFECTIONS. 101

during the progress of dropsy during pregnancy; also *Bryonia* and Hellebore. The indications for the use of *Arsenicum, China* and *Hellebore* are too well known to require repetition here. *Aurum-muriaticum* cured a case of dropsy of one year's standing, first causing a copious secretion of fine clear urine; while *Ononis-spinosa* caused a secretion of turbid urine, of an ammoniacal odor.

Dose.—According to RUECKERT, Arsenicum has been used successfully in six cases of dropsy, generally in the 30th dilution. *Bryonia* in two cases, in the 5th dilution. *Cainca*, in two cases, in the 4th dilution. *Camphor*, in two cases, in the tincture. *China*, in eight cases, in the 4th dilution. *Convolvulus-arolus*, in the 30th potency, is said to have been found very useful in œdematous swellings of all kinds, in dropsy with abdominal obstructions, derangements and debility; it causes liquid stools and profuse flow of urine. *Digitalis*, has been given successfully in the tincture, 4th and 10th dilutions. *Dulcamara*, in two cases, in the tincture, and 7th dilution. *Hellebore*, in twelve cases, in the tincture, 3d, 4th and 30th dilutions. Kali-carb., Lactuca-virosa, Ledum and Lycopodium, each in one case. *Mercurius*, in two cases, in the 1st and 3d dilutions. *Phosphor*, in two cases. *Rhus*, 30th dilution in several cases. Sambucus-*cort-int.*, in one case. And *Stannum-muriat.*, in drop doses of the tincture.

A few words must be added on the treatment of Bright's disease of the kidneys in pregnant females. I claim the credit of being the first to point out a truly homœopathic and epecifically curative remedy, viz.: *Mercurius-corrosivus,* against at least one variety of Bright's disease of the kidneys, (see Homœopathic Examiner, New Series, Vol. 1, p. 285), as long age as the year 1846; (also, see my Treaties on Apoplexy, p. 42). I am sorry to be obliged to admit that *Mercurius-corros,,* will not cure all cases of Albuminuria in pregnant females; perhaps because the disease, in them, aften arises from a mechanical cause, viz: from the pressure of the gravid uterus upon the kidneys, aided somewhat by the unyielding and rigid state of the walls of the abdomen in primaparæ. Emollients applied to the walls of the abdomen, viz: Sweet-oil, Glycerine, aided by the frequent use of warm baths, warm clothing, light diet, &c., &c. may aid in relaxing the abdominal walls, and take off some of the pressure of the womb upon the kidneys. Position may aid somewhat; if possible the anasarcous pregnant female should learn to lie upon her face, or at least upon one or the other side, and never upon her back, at least not for any length of time.

If there be a deficiency of Urea in the urine, *Colchicum* should be used in alternation with *Mercurius-corrosivus*.

FRERICHS has lately given an entirely new explanation of the occurrence of convulsions and coma in Bright's disease in general, and in the dropsical affections of pregnant women. It is well known, that the most sudden and serious attacks of coma and convulsions may occur, when there is but little dropsy, and that there may be a great degree of dropsy, without even drowsiness, much less a tendency to convulsions; yet it very often happens, that drowsiness and dropsy commence and increase together, until complete coma ensues. FRERICHS is even of opinion, that the symptoms of blood-poisoning are not immediately due to the accumulation of urea, or to that of any other of the solid constituents of the urine in the blood, but that they are occasioned by the *Carbonate of Ammonia*, which results from the decomposition of urea within the blood vessels. He supports his opinion by observation and experiment. He states that the air expired by patients who are laboring under symptoms of Uræmic poisoning, (coma, convulsions, &c.) contains an appreciable amount of *Carbonate of Ammonia*, as shown by the restoration of the color of reddened litmus paper, which has been moistened and placed before the mouth and nose; and by the fumes which appear when a rod dipped in Muriatic-acid is placed in the current of expired air. The quantity of *Carbonate of Ammonia* in the expired air bears, he says, a proportion to the intensity of the symptoms. He also states, that the *blood* in the same circumstances contains Carbonate of Ammonia, which is sometimes so abundant as to be detected by the sense of smell, and to produce effervescence on the addition of Muriatic-acid.

In addition to these observations, FRERICHS gives the result of some experiments, which he performed on dogs. After injecting *Urea* into the veins of dogs, whose kidneys had been previously extirpated, he found that the animal remained free for some time (an hour, or more) from the symptoms of poisoning. But after an interval, varying from one hour and a quarter to eight hours, they became restless and vomited, and then were seized with convulsions, followed by drowsiness and stupor

Ammonia was detected in the expired air *simultaneously* with the commencement of the convulsions; and after death, the blood and the contents of the stomach contained large quantities of Ammonia.

In another series of experiments, a solution of *Carbonate of Ammonia* was injected into the blood of the dogs; Convulsions came on immediately, and often were very violent, but they were soon succeeded by drowsiness and stupor. The expired air was at the some time charged with *Carbonate of Ammonia,* and continued so for more than an hour, when the *exhalation* of Ammonia gradually ceased, and consciousness was restored. A fresh injection of *Carb. Ammon.* during the period of stupefaction brought on a recurrence of convulsions with vomiting, and an involuntary passage of urine and fæces. After the lapse of five or six hours the Ammonia again disappeared, and the dog's consciousness and vivacity returned.

JOHNSON says, these experiments are certainly in favor of FRERICH's notion that the *Carbonate of Ammonia, which results from the decomposition of Urea, is the poisonous agent in producing stupor, coma and convulsions,* and *not the* urea itself; and this being the case, it ceases to be surprising, that a large accumulation of urea in the blood may sometimes be unassociated with any symptom of Uræmic poisoning. In order to account for the decomposition of Urea in some cases of Bright's disease, and not in others, FRERICHS assumes the presence of some peculiar ferment in the former cases, which is not present in the latter; but he has no knowledge of the nature of this supposed ferment.

If these suppositions of FRERICHS be true, the use of Hartshorn and smelling salts should be rigidly kept from 'those females, especially when in their first pregnancy, who have any dropsical symptoms or tendencies. The antidotes of Carb. Ammonia may also prove useful, such as Vinegar, Lemon- and Orange-juice and Citric-acid, which convert the Carbonate into the non-poisonous citrate of Ammonia. Or the fumes of Muriatic-acid may be inhaled, which will convert the Carbonate into the non-injurious Muriate of Ammonia; or dilute Muriatic, or Nitric-acid may be given internally, to convert the free Carbonate into the Muriate or Nitrate of Ammonia.

The convertion of urea into Carbonate of Ammonia is quite easy; according to LEHMANN, if organic matters, either putrefying, or capable of undergoing putrefaction be mixed with an aqueous solution of Urea, the latter is soon converted into Carbonic-acid and Ammonia. Also, on heating Urea very slowly it becomes converted into a white glistening body, Carbonic-acid and Ammonia being evolved during the process.

Again, at a temperature a little above 120°, Urea beings to develop Ammonia and to change into Cyamonic-acid; when rapidly heated it yields Cyanic-acid. Hence, in some stages of Bright's Disease, Hydrocyanic-acid may be formed in the blood, and the antidotes for this poison be required

DROPSY OF THE BELLY.—These cases are almost always examples of acute or inflammatory dropsy; they seldom occur till the latter months of pregnancy; the pulse is apt to be quick, with some fever and pain, but there is often very little tenderness; fluctuation is soon very evident, and there is unusual enlargement of the abdomen for the period of pregnancy; the stomach is sometimes disordered, the skin dry and the urine scanty. It is generally preceded by some swelling of the feet and ankles; it is apt to be followed by troublesome cough, difficult respiration, restless nights, frequent starting during sleep, unpleasant dreams, and inabiliy to remain long in the resumbent posture.

Treatment.—HARTMANN regards *Hellebore* as the most important remedy; next China; also Ferrum-aceticum. Also *Digitalis, Colchicum, Scilla* and *Dulcamara*. He has seen good effects from *Euphorbium, Cyparissius* and from *Solanum-nigrum; Prunus-spinosa,* Ledum and Arsenicum deserve attention.

CONVULSIONS.

THESE are generally supposed to be of three kinds, 1st: the nervous or hysteric; 2d, the epileptic; and 3d, the apoplectic.

The *Hysteric convulsions* are most common during the early months of pregnancy; they may be brought on by want of sleep, excessive fatigue, disordered digestion, or in fact by any irritation of body or mind.

CONVULSIONS.   105

The *Epileptic convulsions* are rare; seventy-nine cases only occurred in 38,306 of labor, or 1 in about 485. The majority of these cases are connected with albuminuria, they are apt to be preceded by a peculiar and intense pain in the forehead, severe pain in the stomach, and by a tumid state of the face and hands. Under allopathic treatment forty-two monthers were lost out of one hundred and fifty-two cases, or more than one-fourth.

Apoplectic convulsions seldom or never occur except towards the termination, or after the conclusion of labor, they are generally caused by the stress upon the blood vessels of the brain during the severe forcing labor-pains; they differ from the other varieties by there being but little convulsion; the body and limbs are thrown about for a short time, and then the patient lies in a comatose state; there is little or no distortion of the face, and no frothing at the mouth; the muscles are flaccid and powerless; the breathing stertorous; there is no return of intelligence, and rarely any repetition of the paroxysm.

Treatment.—Dr. WIELOBYCKI reports eleven cases; viz: one case treated successfully by bloodletting, cold to the head, calomel, enemetas and blisters; another by bloodletting, Morphine, brandy and Ammonia; a third, by cold to the head, and weak coffee; a fourth, by Hyosciamus 3d dilution, Coffea 3d and Opium 2d; a fifth, by cold to the head, Nux 4th dilution, and Aconite 5th; a sixth, by Chamomilla 1st dilution, Aconite 4th and Bellad, 6th; a seventh, by a cup of black Coffee, Cicuta 9th and Aconite 6th; an eighth, by Chamomilla 2d and Hyosciamus 3d; a ninth, by Opium, Secale, Soffea and Hyosciam.; a tenth, by Ignatia and Mercurius-solubilis; the eleventh, by Pulsat., Secale and Opium.

He advises warm injections, and *Nux* if the convulsions are connected with obstinate constipation; *Aconite,* if the skin be hot and dry; *Bryonia,* if the abdomen be tender, with full pulse and perspiration; if there be flatulence, and diarrhœa with tenesmus, *Chamomilla, Mercurius* and *Hyosciamus;* if there be difficulty of urination, with coldness and pallor of the face, *Pulsatilla;* if the face be livid, purple and warm, *Belladonna;* if there be a tendency to stupor, with stertorous breathing, or a state of incoherent wandering, *Opium,* which will render the mind clear and calm, with a corresponding improvement of the other symptoms. *Hyosciamus*, when there is an agitated or ruffled state of the nervous system, with an over-active state of the vascular; it acts like a charm, soothing and stilling the nervous system, while the labor goes on progressively. If the labor pains are deficient, they may be aroused by *Secale* or *Pulsatilla*. (See Brit. Journ. of Homœopathy.)

HARTMANN recommends *Opium, Laurocerasus, Stramonium, Bellad., Hyosciamus* and Aconite as the principal remedies.

Laurocerasus, when the convulsion comes on very suddenly, either before or during parturition, attended with tetanic spasms and loss of consciousness, interrupted by violent convulsions, every ten or fifteen minutes, with feeble, hurried and scarcely perceptible pulse.

A few strong doses of *Opium* will often postpone the attacks, and thus afford time for the vital powers to react effectually against the disease. It acts very promptly after bloodletting, and must be repeated not only after every attack of convulsion, but also when there is the least indication of a return.

VARICOSE VEINS.

A dilatation of the veins of the legs, followed by a thickening of their coats, consequent upon the arrest of the ascending column of blood, is a very frequent accompaniment of pregnancy.

They are most frequent on the leg below the knee, but the veins of the thighs are apt to be involved; more rarely the veins of the labia majora, the vagina, and even of the os-uteri become varicose. When the womb is more inclined to one side of the body than the other, then one limb will be affected, whilst the other retains its natural condition.

Treatment.—Arsenicum,, Pulsatilla and *Ferrum-aceticum* have been recommended. *Lycopodium* has improved the varices of pregnant females; and *Fluoric-acid* has reduced by one-half, the numerous varicose veins of some aged persons.

PAIN AND TENSION OF THE BREAST.

Some patients complain of a pricking, or of acute pain in one or both breasts; the pain may be constant, or recur in paroxysms, or even periodically; in most cases there is no fever, the skin is cool and pulse quiet, although the excess of pains may cause sleeplessness and want of appetite; but in others, the pulse becomes quick, skin hot, and even delirium may set in, when the agony is great.

Treatment.—Bryonia is regarded as the most important remedy; if there be erysypelatous redness, heat and hardness, *Bellad.* and *Hepar-sulph.* will be required, or *Mercurius.*

ABORTION.

When this happens before the twentieth day, it has been termed, *Ovular abortion;* before the sixth week, *Miscarriage;* before the third month, *Embryonic abortion;* from the third to the sixth month, Fœtal abortion; any time after the sixth month, *Premature* birth; moles hydatids, &c., are called *False births.*

Abortion are much more frequent during the first two or three months of pregnancy, than at any other time, owing to the feeble attachments of the embryo to the womb; women with profuse menstruation, and those with dysmennorrhœa, are very apt to abort, at what should be a regular menstrual period; especially those females who are subject to severe pain and suffering during the menstrual period, continual bearing-down, and a sense of weight and dragging during menstruation, and also during urination and defecation, particularly if they also have pains about one or both ovaries.

Another cause of abortion is too great *rigidity* of the uterine fibres, and an *unyielding* state of the walls of the womb, thus opposing too great a resistance to the dilatation, which the orgar ought to experience; this is apt to lessen after several abortions; and hence in the *postponing* type of abortion, after it is repeated several times at an advance period, the woman finally goes her full time after the fourh or fifth pregnancy.

A third cause of abortion is feebleness and relaxation of the neck of the womb; a state which Desormeaux has frequently found to exist in some females—this, especially if connected with excessive contractibility and irritability of the womb, is apt to lead to the *anticipating* type of abortion, in which miscarriage occurs each time at an earlier, and still earlier period of time.

WHITEHEAD places great stress upon disease of the neck of the womb as causing abortion; in three hundred and seventy-eight cases, there was disease of the neck in two hundred and seventy-five; the cause was obscure in twenty-nine cases; there was vascular congestion in fifteen cases; constipation of the bowels in three cases; retroversion of the womb in three; placenta prævia in eight, &c. In the majority of these cases, purulent, yellowish, or sanious leucorrhœa was present, as a symptom of ulceration of the neck of the womb.

Abortion is chiefly dangerous from the flowing, which may not only take place at the time, but which may become constant and exhausting even after the delivery of the fœtus, owing to the irritation exerted by the retained membranes, and afterbirth. They should be carefully examined for, and removed.

Treatment.—*Calcarea* has been recommende, when the patient is plethoric, subject to profuse menstruation, leucorrhœa pains in the breasts, colics, pains in the loins. sick-headache rush of blood to the head and chest, &c.

Belladonna is the best remedy, when the above symptoms become more urgent, and immediately threatening, especially if bearing-down-pains set in.

Sabina, is the most homœopathic remedy, when females naturally subject to profuse menstruation, have the premonitory symptoms of abortion, and a little bright red blood has even made its appearance.

Sepia is best suited, when there is an abundant leucorrhœa, the patient being feeble, sad, melancholic, inclined to perspire easily, and being very subject to uterine colics.

Secale is the most homœopathic remedy, when the patient has previously been subject to painful menstruation. and severe forcing pains have already set in.

DISEASES OF PARTURITION.

FALSE LABOR.

WHEN called to a woman apparently in labor, tne accoucheur should first endeavor to ascertain whether she has really attained her full time, so as not to encourage a premature labor, which might be prevented If the neck of the womb is not entirely effaced but still retains a certain degree of length, and is hard and resistent; if the intervals during the pains are not regular in their course, duration and return; and the belly has not yet sunk down, then the physician should endeavor to arrest this premature or false labor by rest of body and mind, and soothing treatment.—CAZEAUX.

There is another occurrence sometimes witnessed in the latter weeks of gestation, which may place the most skilful practitioner in default, viz, what has been designated as *False Labor*, in which some women after having nearly reached their full term experience the true pains and contractions; the pains are regular, the membranes bulge out, and the mouth of the womb dilates; at times these pains last from four to six hours, and then go off; in others, the false labor is kept up for several hours, then passes off, and returns again every evening perhaps for one, or two weeks.

Treatment.—Pulsatilla and Opium are the principal remedies; but constipation, flatulence, acidity, &c. should be obviated.

TREMBLINGS, AND CHILLS.

SOME nervous women are troubled with trembling and chills in the very commencement of their labor, and which are sometimes sufficiently severe to cause much inquietude. These symptoms often coincide with an unusual rapidity in the dilatation of the neck of the womb, and a speedy delivery. Sometimes these shiverings are renewed during, or immediately after labor, but they rarely or never merit serious attention.

Treatment.—Aconite, Cannabis-indica, and Sumbul are important remedies. Opium, when there is trembling, as if from fright, with quivering or distortion of every muscle, with coldness all over. Agaricus, Cuprum, Ammon.-carb., and Cocculus, deserve attention. Gentiana-lutea, when shuddering like electric shocks proceed from the back, through the whole body, followed by great languor. Veratrum, when there is trembling with anguish about the heart and inclination to faint.

DERANGEMENT OF THE STOMACH, &c.

NAUSEA and vomiting are not uncommon during, or at the commencement of labor; they are regarded as good signs, as their presence is said to indicate that the mouth of the womb is rapidly dilating.

Irritability of the bladder, and of the lower bowels, causing the patient to have an almost constant desire for their evacuation are not uncommon in the beginning of labor. And during the last moments of childbirth, the pressure on the lower part of the rectum, produced by the child's head, creates an urgent desire to empty the bowels; and many women yielding to a mistaken modesty, then wish to rise and retire to the water-closet; others, may seize that opportunity to let the child drop upon the floor in the hopes of sacrificing is life. It would of course be exceedingly imprudent to comply with their demands, espeially as the desire is often illusory, particularly in those cases in which the bowels have been fully emptied shortly before the commencement of labor. CAZEAUX once had a patient who was delivered upon the close-stool, without being able to rise, and he not able to afford any assistance to mother or child.

As is well known, a small quantity of fæcal matter often escapes from the rectum during parturition; but if meconium escape from the child during labor, in any other presentation, than a breach one, it is always an unfavourable sign, as it usually indicates a state of suffering of the child, generally from compression of the cord, and consequent congestion of the brain and lungs, followed by relaxation of the sphincters.

Treatment.—Ipecac., Pulsat., and Hydrocyanic-acid are the best remedies against excessive nausea; Bellad., Opium and Stramonium, or Ipecac. against tenesmus of the bowel; Cannabis, against irritability of the bladder. Pressure on the cord should be removed, when there is expulsion of meconium.

NERVOUSNESS.

Many women suffer excessively from nervous agitation and excitement during some one, or all the stages of labor; they feel their pains acutely lose their self-control, and lament in the most heart-rending manner.

Treatment.—In these, and in very difficult and tedious cases, Chloroform is the only reliable remedy. It unquestionably diminishes the duration of labor, by relaxing the parts, soothing the nervous system, and checking the irregular and spasmodic pains which retard the proper expulsive efforts. It takes away the anguish and distress which often proceed from an extremity of suffering almost beyond human endurance; and saves the practitioner and friends from witnessing those struggles and that agony which often almost unnerves them. It diminishes the shock of labor upon the system in general so that the patient often appears quite refreshed, and almost unaffected by the powerful efforts she has made.

With the aid of Chloroform the duties of the practitioner become easy; every manipulation and assistance can be rendered promptly and efficiently, as his feelings and attention are not occupied by cries and groans, struggles and agonies which time alone can relieve, without the aid of Chloroform.

A severe and prolonged fainting fit is the only serious evil to be expected from the use of Chloroform; but that must be attended to in the most prompt and effectual manner; those women who are very apt to faint, especially if their health is naturally delicate, should not insist upon the use of Chloroform.

SLOWNESS, OR FEEBLENESS OF THE CONTRACTIONS.

According to Cazeaux a slowness or feebleness of the contractions of the womb may occur at the very commencement of labor, and persist throughout its whole course.

Treatment.—According to Cazeaux we generally can only

encourage the patient to have patience, and support her strength with broth, claret or some other weak wine and water. Zincum and Cuprum in alternation, at intervals of five or ten minutes; or Zincum and Argentum, or Platina may prove useful. Many homœopathic physicians place great reliance upon Pulsatilla; while Secale, Nux, Ignatia and Angustura deserve attention. Pressure should also be made upon the vaginal surface of the Perinæum.

A. In some cases the feebleness of the pains is owing to excessive distention of the womb, either from the presence of an unusually great quantity of waters, or from the presence of twins. This over-distention renders the walls of the womb much thinner than usual, and lessens their power of contraction; consequently the pains though feeble and only returning at distant and irregular intervals, leave the patient in a state of anxiety and continual suffering.

Treatment.—In these cases an early and artificial rupture of the membranes is the most important step; to be followed by the use of proper medicines, if necessary.

B. In other cases the slowness and feebleness of the pains may depend upon general plethora, or local congestion of the womb. The pains are at first quite energetic, but soon diminish both in frequency and intensity; the womb and vagina are fuller and more heated than common; the breathing may be labored; the pulse hard and full; the face flushed; and the pains very irregular both in force and frequency.

Treatment.—Aconite is the most important remedy; Veratrum-viride and Digitalis, deserve attention.

C. Or there may be debility or inertia of the womb itself, though the patient may otherwise be perfectly healthy, and the other muscles of the organism be endowed with their usual energy.

Treatment.—Secale is supposed to be the only reliable remedy. In all these cases the method of my friend DR. BOLLES, consisting in making decided pressure upon the inner surface of the perinæum, in imitation of the pressure of the child's head, is a most efficient and valuable mode of relieving feebleness of the contractions, and inertia of the womb.

RELAXATION, OR SUSPENSION OF THE PAINS.

It is not at all unusual to find a labor which has been progressing favorably, to become at once arrested, and the pains which had been strong and frequent, diminish or even cease altogether.

A. Any vivid moral impression; the reception of exciting news; injudicious remarks, or discussions in the lying-in chamber; or the presence of a disagreeable person may produce this effect.

Treatment.—*Pulsatilla, Secale,* and pressure upon the perinæum are the most important agents; tickling, or irritating the os-uteri may be employed; or frictions over the region of the womb; and the patient may be allowed to get up and walk about.

B. The occurrence of some other and violent distress or pain may suspend the uterine contractions, such as distressing and repeated vomitings; sharp pains or cramps in the muscles of the back, belly or legs; gripings in the bowels; pains and cramps from the pressure of the child's head on the sacral nerves.

Treatment.—Ipecae., Bellad., Colocynth, &c. may be used with advantage.

IRREGULARITY OF THE PAINS.

According to Cazeaux, the pains may be irregular in their progress, or they may be partial in their operation.

In the *first* variety there is no complete and perfect interval between the pains; they are continuous, but much increased in paroxysms, during which the sufferings are intolerable.

In the *second* variety only a portion of the womb contracts; sometimes it is only the fundus, or one of the angles, or some part of the body of the womb contracts spasmodically, while the remainder scarcely does so at all; but still, the pains are no less severe than if the whole organ were involved; on the contrary, they are often more so, although it is easy to ascertain by ventral and vaginal examinations that the child does not advance at all.

After a while the woman is apt to fall into a state of extreme agitation; she weeps and becomes despondent; very often her pulse becomes frequent and feverish; her face red and flushed; skin hot; mind confused, and the limbs convulsively contracted; the whole forming a state, which has been termed *Uterine tetanus.*

Treatment.—Opium is the most reliable remedy, although Secale, Nux, Pulsatilla, and Ignatia are more homœopathic.

TOO RAPID DELIVERY.

Occasionally we meet with cases in which the child is delivered too rapidly, and such excessive rapidity of labor is apt to be repeated at each successive confinement. This peculiarity has been found to be hereditary in certain families for three or four generations in succession; and it has been supposed to be most common in those females whose menstruation is difficult and painful, the patient being tormented every month with violent colicky pains; it is supposed that this irritability of the womb, will render her liable to excessive and energetic contractions during child-birth.

In these cases the pains are quite strong at the commencement of labor, they are very painful, last a long time, and are separated by short intervals; the patient can not resist the inclination to bear down, and, and forcibly contract the muscles of her body; she is excited and irritable, her head hot, face red and puffed up; pulse full and quick.

In many instances one pain has scarcely terminated before another begins, and sometimes the womb seems in a state of almost permanent contraction until the child is born.

Treatment.—Secale is the most homœopathic remedy, but Bellad, Conium, Strammonium and Chloroform deserved attention.

CONTRACTION AND RIGIDITY OF THE VULVA.

The rigidity of the external parts of generation is frequently observed in women who do not become pregnant until late in life, and also in very muscular girls who are stout and plethoric.

Most commonly the narrowness and rigidity gradually give way; but often there are some slight or severe lacerations of the vagina, or posture commissure. It is not at all unusual in muscular women, in their first child-bed, to find the labor progress very regularly at first, the head of the child passing out of the mouth of the womb, and descending well down upon the perinæum, where its farther progress is at once arrested by the excessive rigidity of that part.

In some instances the uterine pains grow weaker and weaker, and finally cease altogether; in others, the pains are kept up as strong and vigorous as at the commencement of labor, and yet they are unable to overcome the resistance of the perinæum.

Treatmnt.—Stibium, Conium and Tabacum are the remedies most frequently used. The application of cloths wrung out in hot water, may be tried; also the free use of Sweet-Oil, Glycerine, simple Cerate, Muton-suet, &c.

ŒDEMA OF THE LABIA AND THROMBUS.

Dropsical swelling of the external genitals has already been alluded to (see page 98). It can be relieved speedily by making one or several punctures with a lancet into the swollen parts.

Thrombus is the effusion of blood into the external genital parts; the vaginal veins are apt to become enlarged during pregnancy, and one or the other of them may give way during the latter months, or during labor, especially when the head or breach of the child is about to clear the vulva.

The development of such a bloody tumor is generally announced by severe pain in the affected part, followed by the rapid formation of a more or less voluminous tumor of one or the other labia. This tumefaction may attain a considerable size, and the quantity of effused blood may be sufficient to weaken the patient.

Treatment.—Arnica, and Millefolium may be used to stop the hæmorrhage; or some styptic application, such as Tannin, Perchloride of Iron, Ice, &c.

RIGIDITY OF THE NECK OF THE WOMB.

In some cases the fibres of the neck of the womb seem to possess an extraordinary degree of resistance, especially in very young girls, or in middle aged women in their first labors; and in premature confinements.

In some cases the neck of the womb is only more irritable than usual; it is then thin, resistent, tough, hot, dry and painful.

Rigidity of the neck is generally attended with severe pain in the loins.

Spasmodic contraction of the neck may be present at the commencement of labor; may be overcome in part, until the waters are discharged, when the neck is apt to contract again spasmodically; even after this is again overcome and the head of the child has passed through the mouth of the womb, the neck may again contract regidly around the neck of the child, and has to be dilated anew to allow the child's shoulders and body to pass.

Treatment.—Stibium, Stramonium and Belladonna are the most important remedies; the latter remedies may be applied locally to the mouth of the womb.

OBLIQUITY OF THE ORIFICE.

The neck of the womb is usually directed somewhat backwards; besides the posterior lip dilates more rapidly than the anterior; hence any excess of these natural procedure will cause the mouth of the womb to look directly towards the sacrum, and in the progress of labor the dilatation of the neck will be very slowe, because the expulsive efforts will be directed against the anterior portion of the cervix, rather than against the mouth of the womb.

Treatment.—The woman should lie in bed even during the early stages of labor; it will also be better for her to lie upon her back, than upon her side; at the proper time the accucueur should hook the anterior lip with his finger, carefully bring it to the centre of the vagina, and retain it there until a new contraction comes on; the head of the child will then probably be forced down into the opening and no longer permit the lip to return to its unnatural position. The labor will then terminate several hours sooner than it otherwise would.

SWELLING OF THE ANTERIOR LIP.

It is not unusual to find the head descending into the cavity of the pelvis, long before the complete dilation of the mouth of the womb, whereby the anterior lip is necessarily compressed between the head of the child and the symphysis pubis, and considerable tumefaction may occur.

Treatment.—The lip should be pushed back during the intervals of the pains if possible; if this cannot be accomplished, and the swelling be very great, tense and black, a number of punctures may be made for the purpose of evacuating the infiltrated liquids. At times, the progress of the child's head may be aided by introducing the finger into the rectum, and pressing against it.

MOLES.

By mole is meant an organized, fleshy, insensible body, generally softish, sometimes hardish, of variable and indeterminate shape, always the result of depraved conception, which after having been begun and developed within the womb, instead of a fœtus, is sooner or later expelled.

These bodies have been called *false germs*, or *embryonal moles*, when they do not remain in the womb more than two or three months, and are covered with the usual envelopes or membranes of the fœtus, within which a transparent or bloody fluid is enclosed, together with some traces of an embryo.

Hydatid moles consist in a degeneration of the placenta, or after-birth, within which there is developed a greater or smaller number of cysts, either separate or united, like the fruit of a bunch of grapes. This kind of mole is very common; often attains a great size; remains for a long time in the womb; and finally is expelled either in mass, or in broken pieces.

The *fleshy mote* does not require particular description.

The recognition of the presence of a mole within the womb is extremely difficult during the early months, because the symptoms are equally characteristic of true pregnancy; the both cases we find: suppression of the menses, swelling of the breasts, enlargement of the figure, disgust, nausea and general derangement of various functions. At a later period, the size of the abdomen is apt to be greater than it is at a corresponding stage of real pregnancy; it is generally more painful, harder, and more equally distended; there is no *baloitement,* and no motion of a child; the weight of the womb seems greater and more fatiguing than when it contains a fœtus; the woman suffers more from pain in the loins, difficult urination and lassitude than she does in an ordinary pregnancy, and often feels somethng like a ball falling about within her as she turns from side to side. The breasts enlarge at first, then shrink and shrivel up; and frequent and irregular attacks of bleeding from the womb are apt to occur. After the lapse of the first five months we can generally decide upon the nature of the case from the absence of the signs of true prgnancy, the presence of local uneasiness, and the recurrence of floodings.

Treatment.—We should generally wait until nature expels the foreign body, and then use the same care and precautions as in ordinary labor. In some cases the use of *Secale* is necessary; in other cases the mouth of the womb must be dilated with the hand, or with the aid *Belladonna*-ointment, and the foreign body removed with the fingers, or instruments. Carbo-vegetabilis, Sulphur, Sabina and Bovista may be used to prevent the growth of moles.

EXTRA UTERINE PREGNANCY.

The commonest form is tubal pregnancy. The abdominal tumor rises out of the pelvis earlier than usual; is found far over to one or the other side; is irregular and modulated in form; and while the motions of the fœtus are readily detected, we find the size and weight of the womb but slightly increased, and the neck of the womb but little shortened. It generally terminates spontaneously before the fifth month, by the rupture of the fallopian tube and escape of the child into the cavity of the abdomen, marked by the occurrence of sudden and acute pain, rapid exhaustion, paleness and syncope; although these may be preceded by labor-pains, dilation of the mouth of the womb, discharge of bloody and glairy mucus from the vagina, and evident contractions in the womb and tumor.

Treatment.—In some cases it may be justifiable to resort to the operation of Gastronomy (CAZEAUX); in case of rupture of the tube, the only hope is in the judicious use of large doses of Opium, as in cases of rupture of the bowels and womb.

DELIVERY OF THE AFTER-BIRTH.

IN a large number of cases, immediately after the birth of the child, the after-birth will be found lying high up in the vagina, but completely within the reach of the accoucheur In a certain number of other cases the detachment of the after-birth and its ejection from the womb into the vagina is effected in the course of fifteen, twenty, or twenty-five minutes, but having passed into the vagina, it sometimes remains there for several hours without causing the least irritation by its presence, nor the least bearing-down effort; on the country, the walls of the vagina will often gradually contract around it and retain it there for an indefinite period.

In all these cases, and they form the greater number, the accoucheur should make but little traction upon the cord, but carefully and gently pass his fingers up until he reach sufficient of the placenta to grasp it and bring it down. If he cannot reach it, some traction may be made upon the cord, pressure should be made on the inner surface of the perinæum, or posterior wall of the vagina, and frictions to the hypogastric region with a cool or cold hand. Some practitioners regard these procedures as unjustifiable; but although the delivery of the after birth may generally be left to the powers of nature without any serious inconvenience, yet it is equally true that it will be delayed a long time in a large number of cases. Now, such delay will not only force the patient to remain in an uncomfortable situation, but so long as the delivery is not completed, she will still consider herself exposd to numerous dangers, and her fears may have an unfavourable influence over her condition.

If the after-birth be entirely retained within the womb, the accoucheur may make pressure on the posterior wall of the vagina, irritate the mouth of the womb gently, use pressure and friction over the lower part of the belly, and allow at least one full hour to elapse after the child is born, before proceeding to more active measures, such as the introduction of the hand into the womb, and the use of Ergot.

Retention of the after-birth from irregular or spasmodic contraction of the womb; or from spasmodic contraction of either the external or internal orifice, hour-glass contraction, or from spasmodic contraction of the whole organ may be relieved by the use of Nux, Ignatia or Secale, or if these fail, by Opium, Bellad, or Stramonium, aided by the usual manipulations of overcoming the stricture by careful introduction of the hand.

Adhesions of the placenta must be carefully overcome by mechanical means; the after-birth should be pealed off, and then removed by the hand. The details are given in every book on midwifery.

HÆMORRHAGE BEFORE, DURING, OR AFTER THE DELIVERY OF THE AFTER-BIRTH.

This is one of the most frequent and at the same time the most terrible of the accidents which complicate the delivery of the after-birth. This accident is frequently developed in the course of a few minutes after the child is born, though sometimes the inertia of the womb is secondary, as it were, not coming on for several hours, or even not until several days after. The womb after having been fully and properly contracted after the birth of the child or delivery of the after-birth, may become relaxed by degrees, and ultimately give rise to a frightful hæmorrhage.

The signs by which the existence of flowing is made out, are easily recognized; but the discharge is sometimes so sudden and profuse that the woman's life is almost immediately seriously endangered. The patient generally complains of a feeling of weight about the stomach; and soon after, a pallor of the face, dimness of vision, smallness of the pulse, debility and fainting are apt to set in.

When the blood appears externally, there is no doubt about the nature of the case; but when the bleeding is internal, and confined to the cavity of the womb, the nature of the case may escape detection, and at least only be recognized when it is too late to remedy it.

The majority of these cases may be prevented by a little care on the part of the accoucheur; as the body of the child is being born, careful pressure should be made upon the body of the womb, by a friend, nurse or assistant; and this pressure should be continued without the least interruption until the bandage is well applied. After delivery the patient should lie perfectly flat, with her thighs stretched out along side of each other, and then be left in silence, and the most absolute rest of body and mind for at least half an hour. As soon after delivery as possible a perfectly clean and warm napkin ssould be applied to the vulva, and the nurse authoritatively instructed to examine it at least every three or five minutes. Thus any unusual flowing will be detected at a very early period. Besides, I always have a bladder, ice, Ergot and Ammonia at hand, in order that it may be used immediately, if necessary. In case of any excessive flowing, the bladder moderately filled with cracked ice should be placed over the womb, on top of the bandage; a small bit of ice may be introduced into the vagina moderately high up; and Secale may be given every three, five, ten or fifteen minutes according to the urgency of the case; if great weakness or fainting set in, Ammonia should be used. I never leave the most favorable and ordinary case of confinement without having Secale already prepared for use, with stringent instructions to the nurse to examine the napkin frequently, and give Secale, Ice, &c. promptly, until I can be recalled.

If the *tampon* be necessary, I prefer Lint dipped in ice-water vinegar and water, or Alum-water, to any other. A coagulum is more readily formed in the meshes of the lint, than in any other material. Linen and Silk generally restrain the hæmorrhage very imperfectly.

According to CAZEAUX, when the physician has been fortunate enough to restrain the flowing, he should still remain with his patient for several hours, carefully watching the character and amount of discharge from the vulve, and occasionally examining the region of the womb in order to detect any unusual increase in size of it.

After a profuse flowing the patient is naturally inclined to sleep, and some persons think it better to prevent her from slumbering too long lest the discharge should return without her knowledge. But sleep restores the exhausted powers, and ought not to be too soon interrupted; but the patient should never be left alone, and the pulse, size of the womb, and quantity of discharge should be frequently examined by the attendant.

Some patients are frequently tormented, after profuse floodings, by vomiting, or nausea and retching; the vomiting may exhaust the patient and cause fainting, during which the flowing may return again.

Treatment.—Ipecac., Pulsat., or Opium may be required.

INVERSION OF THE WOMB

This accident, according to Cazeaux is always attended by symptoms which are serious in proportion to the amount of inversion. The patient not only suffers from pain, but is harassed by a constant desire to urinate, and straining at stool, which are often sufficient to render an inversion complete, which otherwise would only have been partial. The pain then often becomes excruciating, and the frightened sufferer is apt to faint away; the pulse becomes feeble, or almost imperceptible. The symptoms are less severe when there is a simple depression of the base of the womb; they are urgent when the fundus has been forced down through the mouth of the womb, and this is firmly and spasmodically contracted. When there is partial detachment of the placenta there will be more or less flooding; and if there be complete inertia of the womb, the flowing will be frightful; when the after-birth is adherent there will be no discharge.

Inversion may happen in a very rapid labor, especially if the patient happen to be standing while the child is born; it is more frequently produced by pulling upon the cord, in overhasty attempts to deliver the placenta; and has happened when the patient has sat up too soon (within twelve hours) to have her bewels or bladder relieved.

Treatment.—The patient should be placed upon her back, with her hips raised, and the accoucheur should pass his hand into the cavity of the womb, and gently push the fundus up and back. A mere symptomatic treatment of the pains and other symptoms, is worse than useless.

CONVALESCENCE AFTER PARTURITION.

ACCORDING to MURPHY, the activities of the nervous and circulating systems, which were at their maximum of intensity during the progress of child-bright, are reduced to their minimum after delivery. The pulse sinks; chills, more or less severe may set in, so that the patient either complains of feeling cold, or is actually shivering; she also experiences a certain amount of depression, feels exhausted, and occasionally a slight temporary wandering of the mind gives more distinct evidence of the exhaustion of the nervous power.

The first twelve hours which elapse after 'the birth of the child should be essentially hours of repose; and, if by good management the patient is left undisturbed during that, or even a much shorter interval, and obtains some sound and refreshing sleep, it is surprising how quickly she will be refreshed and restored. The mother has forgotten all her sorrows, is cheerful, disposed to talk, and so far as her own feelings are concerned, it seems to her as if she could get up and go about as well as before delivery. In the next interval, say at the end of twenty-foure hours more, a slight change may be observed; a new function, that of lactation is becoming active, and the circulation, which was below par, now rises again to the febrile, or inflammatory standard; some chilliness, thirst and headache, followed by perspiration, are felt; these symptoms finally disappear when the full secretion of milk is established, and no further constitutional disturbance may be observed.

In the *first period,* or that immediately after delivery, the causes of pain, sickness or other disturbance will generally be found in the errors of those, who are in immediate attendance upon the patient; the most perfect repose of the system is required, and much mischief may result, if the patient is kept in a constant state of worry and excitement after her delivery. The accoucheur often has a right to complain of the well-intentioned but too officious kindness of friends, when he finds on his next visit, that his patient has not slept, that her pulse is quick, that she has some headache, and is thirsty. These premonitions of a more decided febrile paroxysm may be unnoticed by the friends or nurse, but often excite alarm to the careful and experienced practitioner. It is not necessary that the patient should have seen too many visitors in order to produce these results; the nurse may very judiciously have expelled all intruders, and so far succeed in keeping her patient quiet, and who would have enjoyed the repose so necessary for her, if unfortunately the nurse herself had not a strong prejudice in favor of making her "clean and comfortable," that is, all the soiled sheets and bed clothes have been forcibly removed, the patient's dress changed, and after this and sundry other things have been done, the nurse consoles herself with the belief that her charge will now sleep comfortably. But delicate women are very susceptible of nervous irritation at this time; if their rest be once disturbed, or their sleep be put astray, they remain wakeful and unrefreshd; presntly the senses become more than usually excited; the noise of their infant, although from another apartment disturbs them; light becomes exceedingly unpleasant to them, and finally, although the nurse carefully darkens the room and closes the bed-curtains, the patient does not sleep; and even if she does fall into a slight dose, it is but momentary, for the slightest noise or whispering awakes her. After some hours, headache will set in, and just as the secretion of milk is fairly commencing, it may be arrested by the presence of an irregular nervous fever, chills occur at irregular intervals; the headache becomes more severe; the pulse becomes frequent and perhaps irregular, and sometimes delirium may set in. A feverish and nervous disturbance of this kind may not be subdued for weeks, and often has its origin in no other cause, than in a little want of knowledge in the management of th patient immediately after her delivery. MURPHY has known a patient to be lifted up, drawn down to the bottom of the bed, then dragged up again, now to one side, and then to the other in this process of changing the bed clothes, who afterwards presented a most alarming train of nervous symptoms, and all this because the nurse insisted upon making her "comfortable."

Too much excitement is not the only risk to which the woman is exposed during this interval. Errors in diet may very easily be committed. After the patient has had a refreshing sleep, she is apt to feel, and thinks that she is perfectly well, and may eat and enjoy whatever she can get hold of. There is therefore sometimes the greatest possible temptation to partake of too hearty food, the mischief of which may not become apparent for some time, viz., until reaction sets in; but when the pulse naturally begins to rise, and the milk to form, the natural febrile paroxysm may be superseded by one of a more decided and serious character.

Treatment.—The chilliness should be met with warm clothing, by some warm tea, or gruel, or milk and water; if it persists, or returns frequently, China or Arsenicum may be given.

If the patient be feverish, restless and nervous, Aconite and Chamomilla may be administered.

If there be much headache with a tendency to delirium, Aconite and Belladonna.

Errors in diet, may be contracted by the use of some gentle laxative medicine, or by Ipecac, or Pulsatilla.

For the treatment of obstinate sleeplessness, see page 96.

Other and frequent consequences of these cleanly and orderly intermeddlings, are the occurrence of severe after pains, or of more or less dangerous floodings. The patient cannot be moved about in this way without disturbing the bandage that was to secure and support the womb. If the patient leave the horizontal posture, and she is often allowed to set bolt upright, the blood will again accumulate in the uterine veins blood is consequently poured into the cavity of the womb, where if it go no farther, and coagulates, will expose the patient to a severe attack of after-pains; but it may not coagulate, but flow away, and produce a most violent and dangerous flooding. The patient is thus exposed to the risk of her life, at a time when every moment of repose is of the highest value to her, and her physician is probably far away from her.

Treatment.—Severe after-pains require the use of Arnica, Belladonna, Strammonium, Secale, or Opium.

For the treatment of flooding, see page 82.

LACTATION MILK-FEVER, &c.

The *second* period of time after parturition is marked by an increase in 'the force and frequency of the pulse; a slight chill, some thirst and perhaps headache: the breasts are becoming distended. If the previous management of the patient has been judicious, or no other causes of disease be present, the patient will pass safely over this period. The distention of the breasts and the natural fever that accompanies it, are relieved chiefly by the child; when the milk flows freely, the fever subsides, and the function of lactation is established; but very slight causes will derange this natural process, such as improper food, agitation of mind, exposure to cold. In some cases the patient has a severe chill, followed by profuse perspiration, forming the so-called milk-fever. In other instances the formation of milk is too rapid, although there is not much fever; still the breasts become tensely distended and painful, presenting a firm unyielding surface to the infant, who cannot grasp the nipple sufficiently to nurse; hence the breasts are not relieved, and inflammation is apt to set in. In another set of cases the secretion of milk may be suspended or suppressed, and the absence of milk is the precursor of some deeper-seated and more distant inflammation, or of puerperal fever itself. Hence the practitioner should be very solicitous that the function of lactation be safely established; if he child is strong enough and healthy, and if the mother be properly managed previously, this object is generally successfully accomplished. But, both local and constitutional causes may throw impediments in the way; the nipple may be badly formed, either too small or too large, or perhaps flattened by the fashionable corset, so as to form a depression in place of a prominence, so that the child cannot properly grasp it. Or it may happen that the extremely delicate skin that covers the nipple is very irritable and easily inflamed, consequently it will not yield to the traction of the child; it gives way at the base of the nipple; fissures are the result; they bleed easily, and in place of a comfort and enjoyment, the nursing of the child becomes 'the greatest source of anguish and distress to the mother. Again, we may meet with cases in which the breasts and nipples are well formed, nevertheless the milk will not flow, because the minute milk-ducts are not free to transmit it; they may be plugged up with a thick tenacious secretion which the child has not sufficient suction-power to remove.

In another class of cases the milk is secreted scantily, and what is extracted contains but little nourishment; the infant, therefore, is never satisfied, and after having obtained what it can it may sleep, exhausted by its effects to draw the breasts; but it is only a momentary dose, for it soon wakes up, becomes feverish, cries constantly, and is ravenously hungry; the mother has no farther supply, her anxiety contributing still more to arrest the secretion; and thus difficulties of no ordinary character arise.

There are also certain constitutions where there is no deficiency of milk in the breasts, but it is of poor or bad quality; the milk may be abundant, but it does not satisfy the child, or possibly it may produce a considerable amount of irritation in the stomach and bowels of the infant; the child may scarcely have obtained a sufficient quantity before it is ejected from the stomach, or if it pass down into the bowels there will soon be evidences of irritation in its passage along the intestines and an exhausting diarrhœa may place the infant in extreme danger of its life; or it may be exposed to all the torments of colic, and its wild screams that cannot be appeased, soon give evidence of the agony it is enduring.—(MURPHY.)

Treatment.—If the flow of milk be excessive, we must reduce the force of the general circulation, and prevent the effects of over-distention of the breasts. Aconite and Antimony are the most important remedies. But Bryonia may be given if the afflux of milk is very considerable and the breasts greatly distended, so as to produce pain and oppression of the chest; it will generally relieve the tumid breasts and check the fever. Still, *Belladonna* may be required if there be violent pains in the head, tendency to delirium, glistening of the eyes, and fever. Warm fomentations skilfully managed so as to maintain an equal temperature around the distended breasts are often most grateful to the patient; and gentle frictions with warm oil over the surface are useful in promoting the absorption of the excess of milk; when the distention and consequent irritation are relieved, the milk which has been arrested will frequently flow quite freely; if it be slow, the breast-pump may be used, or what is still better, another child, older and stronger, may be applied, and will soon reduce the distention. If it should happen that the milk-ducts are much obstructed, even these methods may fail, and some female friend or nurse must be called upon; their stronger powers of suction will soon remove these plugs, and the milk then flows without difficulty. As soon as this excessive distention is once overcome, it does not generally return, provided caution be used in the diet of the patient, and some gentle laxative medicines are given.

When the flow of milk is *deficient* we haeve a far more difficult case to manage; in the first place the babe must be fed artificially, so as to prevent its restlessness. It may then be applied to the mother at longer intervals than usual, twice perhaps in the day, and once at night, so as to allow the milk which is but slowly secreted, time to accumulate. The mother will generally require a more nutritious diet than can usually be given after parturition; and if the deficiency of milk depends upon the exhaustion and diminished sustenance which have been caused by a protracted labor, even stimulant are sometimes necessary; broth or soup may be given, and, with caution, warm negus. It also essential that sufficient rest and sleep be secured the mother; these patients are apt to be particularly restless, because the desire of the mother to nurse her infant is too frequently strong in proportion to her inability to do so; she is unwilling to resign her little charge to the care of another, and becomes anxious, irritable and sleepless. But the more general causes of deficiency of milk would seem to be a lymphatic constitution, a feebleness of arterial action, or of the vital energies; or a general constitutional debility produced by moral causes, depressing mental emotions, or by an unhealthy pregnancy. In these cases, LEADAM says that *Agnus*-castus is the most useful remedy; if the mother is desirious of nursing, and the signs of milk are not apparent in thirty six hours after delivery, the *Agnus* should be given at once; it is also equally useful, when the milk diminishes or disappears without any appreciable cause, or becomes impoverished; Conium and Iodine also deserve attention.

DR. KALLENBACH having noticed that when Assafœtida

plasters had been applied to the pit of the stomach in hysterical females for a long time, they were sometimes followed by swelling of the breasts, from which a milky fluid oozed, gave it internally with success in four cases. LEADAM has found it to materially increase the flow of milk, improve its quality, and cause the child, which before was pining and constantly disturbed by flatulent colics, to thrive and cease crying.

THE USE OF THE BOFAREIA,

("RICINUS COMMUNIS" OF BOTANISTS) AS A MEANS ADOPTED BY THE NATIVES OF THE CAPE DE VERD ISLAND, TO EXCITE LACTATION.

By Dr. J. O. M'WILLIAM, F.R.S., R.N., &c.

While engaged in an official investigation into the nature and history of a yellow fever epidemy, prevailing in the Island of Boa Vista, in the Cape de Verds, during the year 1846, my attention was called to a remedy commonly had recourse to there, and in the other islands of the group, to accelerate and increase the flow of milk from the breasts of childbearing women, in cases where that secretion was tardy in appearing, or deficient in quantity when it did appear.

I also learnt that, on occasions of emergency, this remedy could be successfully applied to a still more important use, namely, to produce milk in the breasts of women who are not childbearing, or who even have not given birth to, or suckled a child for many years.

The leaves of a plant, called, in the language of the country, Bofareira, but which, in reality is the "Ricinus Communis" of botanists, and, occasionally, the leaves of the "Jatropha curcas," both belonging to the natural family *euphorbilaciæ*, are the means by which these interesting if not extraordinary results are produced.

The Bofareira grows in most if not all, the Cape the Verd Islands. That used by the natives for the purposes I have mentioned, is called by them the *white* bofareira, to distinguish it from what appears to be nothing more than a variety of the same species, the *red* bofareira. The *white*, or that which possesses galactagogue qualities, is recognized by the natives by the light green color of the stem of the leaf, whilst the leaf stem of the *red* is of a purplish red hue. The latter plant is carefully avoided, as it is said to be a powerful irritant, and, if applied as it occasionally has been, by mistake, for the *white*, it produces an immediate and often immoderate flow of the menses.

In cases of childbirth, when the appearance of the milk is delayed (a circumstance of not unfrequent occurrence in those islands) a decoction is made by boiling well a handful of the *white* Bofareira in six or eight pints of spring water. The breasts are bathed with this decoction for fifteen or twenty minutes. Part of the boiled leaves are then thinly spread over the breasts, and allowed to remain until all moisture has been removed from them by evaporation, and probably, in some measure, by absorption. This operation of fomenting with the decoction and applying the leaves, is repeated at short intervals until the milk flows upon suction by the child, which it usually does in the course of few hours.

On occasions where milk is required to be produced in the breasts of women who have not given birth to or suckled a child for years, the mode of treatment adopted is as follows:—

Two or three handfuls of the leaves of the Ricinus are taken and treated as before. The decoction is poured, while yet boiling, into a large vessel, over which the woman sits so as to receive the vapor over her thighs and generative organs, cloths being carefully tucked around her so as to prevent the escape of the steam. In this position she remains for ten or twelve minutes, or until the decoction cooling a little, she is enabled to bathe the parts with it, which she does for fifteen or twenty minutes more. The breasts are then similarly bathed, and gently rubbed with the hands; and the leaves are afterwards applied to them in the manner already described. These several operations are repeated three times during the first day. On the second day, the woman has her breasts bathed, the leaves applied, and the rubbing repeated three or four times. On the third day, the sitting over the steam, the rubbing, and the application of the leaves to, with the fomentation of, the breasts, are again had recourse to. A child is now put to the nipple, and, in a majority of instances, it finds an abundant supply of milk.

In the event of milk not being secreted on the third day, the same treatment is continued for another day, and if then there still be want of success, the case is abandoned, as the person is supposed not to be susceptible to the influence of the Bofareira. Women with well-developed breasts are most easily affected by the Bofareira. When the breasts are small and shrivelled, the plant then is said to act upon the uterine system, bringing on the menses, if their period be distant, or causing their immoderate flow if their advent be near.

Exposure to cold is carefully avoided by persons who are being brought under the influence of the Bofareira. They scrupulously abstain from wetting with cold water either the hands or the feet.

Maria, a dark mulatto woman, with woolly hair, thirty years of age, tall, stout, and well-formed; menstruating regularly; the mother of three children, the youngest of whom was three years old, and had been weaned when under the age of one year, was brought before me by Dr. Almeida, of Boa Vista, on the morning of the 30th of June, 1846, for the purpose of being submitted to the action of the Bofareira. She stated that when her child was weaned, every trace of milk disappeared from her breasts in the course of a few days. I could not detect any sign of pregnancy. The breasts were like those of negro women in general who have borne children, pendulous and flabby. No sign of milk was given out from them upon careful expression of the nipple.

The baths, fomentations, the application of the leaves, friction, suction, &c., were adopted in the manner and order I have already described. On the second day there was a slight oozing of serous-looking milk from the nipples; with slight increase of size in the areolar portion of the breast. On the third day the milk was increased in quantity, and less watery. On the morning of the fourth day there was evident enlargement of the lower part of the mamma, and milk flowed abundantly upon the application of a child to the nipple.

The use of the Bofareira in cases of childbirth, to accelerate the flow of milk, is common, but comparatively rare as a means of procuring a wet-nurse. Some instances of the latter kind occurred, in consequence of the death of mothers with children at the breast during the progress of the Boa Vista epidemy of 1845—46, which decimated a population consisting almost wholly of blacks, with a few Europeans—Portuguese and English—and a small proportion of mixed negro and European blood.

Generally, however, this use of the Bofareira is seldom called for. Death in childbirth, or prolonged illness after parturition, sometimes requires a kind relative to charitable neighbor, who for the safety of the offspring, places herself under the influence of the Bofareira.

The son of a wealthy landed proprietor of San Nicolao (well known to my friend, Mr. George Miller, of that island,) a remarkably hale and robust-looking man, was wet-nursed by a woman who gave him milk produced by the bofareira. The nurse in this instance had borne two children in early life. Her husband had died shortly after the birth of her second child; she lived in a state of virtuous widowhood, and it was *many* years after the death of her husband that she so generously submitted herself to the bofareira, and nursed the infant in question.

Consul-General Rendall, of the Cape de Verds, informs me that a lady, a native of Boa Vista, now residing at San Antonio, and the wife of one of the foreign consuls, had a daughter in 1843. "Having very little milk," says Mr. Consul Rendall, "she caused an old female servant to be prepared with the bofareira, and to act as wet-nurse, which she did in the most satisfactory manner, having plenty of good milk, although she had not had a child for ten years previously. The child is now (March, 1847) a healthy one, and well-grown. "In short," continues M. Rendall, "women who use the bofareira are in two or three days in order sufficient to nurse the child of a queen."

I have not been able to ascertain, from personal observation, or from any very accurate information, what effect the bofareira has upon virgins, or upon those who, although they have not borne children, are nevertheless not virgins. As regards the latter class, however, an intelligent native midwife assured my most able and observant friend, Mr. George Miller, of San Nicolao, that the effect of the administration of the bofareira is much the same upon them as upon them as upon childbearing women.

In some cases, but rarely, the decoction of the bofareira is taken internally, with a view of assisting the action of its external application.

I regret not having been informed of the alleged difference in the action of the white and red bofareiras, while I was at the Cape de Verds, 'that I might have examined the latter plant upon the spot.

The seeds of each plant were, however, kindly forwarded to me by Mr. George Miller, and Sir William Hooker most readily and obligingly examined them. Sir William, in a note to me, says, "What you remark as red bofareira and as white bofareira, are both, not only of the genus 'ricinus,' but also of one and the same species—viz., ricinis communis, the common palma Christi, or castor-oil plant. In our gardens, as well as abroad, the plants vary, and your two plants vary a little in the form and size of the seed, and especially in the color, but they are one and the same species."

It is thus evident that the white and and red bofareiras, if they differ at all, can only be varieties of the same species. It is known, however, that certain varieties of other plants, as thyme, mint, &c., do yield different properties, and such may be the case with the bofareiras.

I have thus stated all the facts that have come to my knowledge regarding 'this galactagogue of the Cape de Verds, which I consider to be well worthy of a fair trial in this country. Should its action in our more temperate regions be similar to that which it exerts within the tropics, an interesting field of inquiry will be opened, as regards ts hygienic, medical, medico-legal, and other relations.

These, however, are points, the consideration of which had better be reserved until it has been determined, by experiment, how far the bofareira can be successfully introduced into the practice of this country.

Note.—Dr. Tyler Smith, to whom I showed my paper before my visit to Edinburgh, has written to inform me that he has in several cases tried the bofareira in the manner described by me; and he assures me that the effects of the plant grown in this country fully bear out the facts I have detailed respecting the use of this plant in the Cape de Verd Islands.—*Lancet,* September 7th, 1850, *p.* 294.

GALACTAGOGUE AND EMMENAGOGUE EFFECTS OF THE LEAVES OF THE BOFAREIRA, (RICINUS COMMUNIS, OR PALMA CHRISTI.)

By. Dr. Tyler Smith.

[Dr. Smith states, that being struck by the facts related in Dr. Mc William's paper, and learning for the first time that the plant is no other than the ricinus communis, which grows as an annual plant in this country, he determined to ascertain by Dr. Mc Willianms' wish, whether the plant when growing in our latitudes, preserves its remarkable properties of stimulating the mammary glands. Dr. Smith says:]

In directing the use of the Bofareira leaves, which I have procured from the Botanical Gardens at Chelsea, Kew, and the Regent's Park, I have followed as nearly as possible the description of Dr. Mc William, with the exception of the application of the steam of the decoction to the generative organs. The following are the cases in which the agent has been used under my directions.

The following case was conducted by Mr. C. Stillman, one of the house-surgeons of Queen Adelaide's Lying-in-Hospital.

Case I.—Mrs. C., twenty-four years of age, rather tall and thin, mother of two children, had weaned the last about six weeks, and had still a little milk, of a very thin, serous character, left in the breasts. She commenced the use of the Bofareira, on the morning of Wednesday, August 21st, by bathing the left breast only, with a strong decoction of the leaves. The leaves themselves were afterwards applied to this breast. In the evening, she repeated the bathing; after which she perceived, on squeezing the nipple, that her milk, which was at first thin and watery, had now become quite thick. After repeating the application on Thursday the 22d, she felt throbbing pains in the breast, accompanied by sickness and pains in the back, which she described as being like after-pains, and the areola surrounding the left nipple had become much darker than the right; the glandular follicles were also larger than in the nipple which had not been under the influence of the Bofareira. The difference between the two breasts was very marked. Having at this time no more leaves, she was unable to continue the application. On the following day, a fresh supply of the leaves was obtained, and she again bathed her left breast as before. After two applications, the *catamenia* appeared before the regular time and the fomentations were not afterwards continued.

Case II.—Mrs. H., mother of four children, her youngest child aged one year and five months, had been weaned more than six months. During the latter months of lactation, she had little milk; the breasts were small, and the nipples contracted. Before applying the Bofareira, the breasts were carefully examined, to learn if they still contained any traces of milk. After much trial, she could squeeze from her left breast the smallest points of serum from the mouths of two or three of the galactophorous ducts, as is the case with most women who have sucked; but from the right breast not a trace of moisture could be expressed. The Bofareina was used night and morning for four days, by bathing with the decoction, and the application of he hot leaves to both breasts, in the manner described by Dr. Mc William. After the second application, thick milk, like the colostrum, could be squeezed from both nipples, the breasts were considerably swollen, the glands in the axillæ were also painful, and pains extended down the arms. There were, in fact, in this case, all the symptoms present, in a minor degree, which are usually observed in the establishment of the milk after parturition. Mrs. H. had also distinct periodical pains in the back and abdomen, which she compared to after-pains. A leucorrhœal discharge was also produced. At the end of the fourth day, milk flowed so freely into a breast-pump, that there was no doubt she could have suckled a child; but at this point the application of the Bofareia was omitted, and the milk has since gradually disappeared.

Case III.—Mrs. D., a married lady, without family, hearing of the use of the Bofareira in the last case, wished it tried upon herself. As there was no possibility of injury she supplied with some of the leaves, and proceeded to use it. The application, and the use of the decoction, produced swelling of the breasts, pain in the back, and an increase of a leucorrhœal discharge, to which she is subject; but there was no appearance of milk in the breasts. At the time of using the Bofareira, the catamenial discharge had ceased about a week.

Case IV.—M. L., a young woman, who had ben delivered three weeks, but whose milk, though profuse, was so poor as to be little more than serum, used the Bofareira three times. under its use the secretion from the breasts became markedly thicker; but the child was unfortunately attacked with diarrhœa, and it was not thought advisable to continue the use of this agent longer.

Case V.—L. M., a young woman, mother of one child, but who had weaned her infant about a year and a half, applied the Bofareira in the form of decoction and poultices two or three times; but the pain and swelling were so considerable, that she refused to go on with it. She had a little serum in the breasts, at the time when the use of the Bofareira was commenced. The secretion speedily became milky. This patient had a leucorrhœa, which had been present, ever since the weaning; and the uterine and vaginal irritation, upon which the leucorrhœa depended, had kept up, in all probability, the serous secretion from the breasts, which is common enough in leucorrhœal cases.

Since the foregoing cases occurred, I have used the remedy in a case of scanty menstruation of a remarkable kind. Owing to exposure to marsh malaria, some years ago, the patient had scarcely a sign of colored discharge at the usual catamenial periods. She use the infusion of the leaves of the red Bofareira at the date of her period, applying the infusion and leaves to the breasts, and the vapor to the genitals, with the effect of producing, in two days, a considerable flow of the catamenia. From the effects in this case, and in one of the cases already related, the Bofareira, promises to be of considerable value as a direct emmenagogue; at all events the cases in which I have tried it, show that the plant does not lose its efficacy in this climate. I hope that, in America and other parts in which the plant is common, perennial instead of annual, extensive trials of its efficacy both as an emmenagogue and a galactagogue, will be made.—*London Journal of Medicine, Oct.* 1850, p. 951.

SORE-NIPPLES.

ACCORDING to MURPHY, *the local cause* that chiefly interferes with nursing, is the extreme tenderness of the nipples, or the fissures, or so called "sore-nipples". If attention be paid to the breasts before delivery, if the nipples be prepared or hardened by astringents, weak brandy, Arnica- or Alum-water, there will be less risk of accidents afterwards. Still, this process of hardening may fail, or it may not have been tried; and then, as soon as the child is applied to the breast it causes great pain; inflammation follows, and a crack, or fissure in the nipple is the consequence. From the moment tris happens the patient's miseries begin; every time the child is applied, the wound is opened and bleeds; the inflammation increases, the nipple swells and becomes painful, even when the child is not drawing upon it; but the pain becomes intolerable when the child nurses; and thus a very slight inflammation in the beginnnig may soon become so severe and obstinate as to require weeks before it is subdued.

The treatment of sore nipples is the treatment of inflammation; and the first and most important point is the prevention of the fissure. It is here that the watchfulness and intelligence of the nurse is of the utmost importance. It is not usual for physicians to examine the breasts and nipples of his child-bed patients every day, tlthough there are many good reasons why he should do so, especially if he has the least reason to suspect any deficiency or tenderness of the nipples, or inflammation. The nurse has daily and hourly opportunities for observation; if there be any great pain, unusual swelling, or redness of the nipple, she must necessarily soon observe it, and always should give timely notice to the physician. But many women have an unreasonable and foolish disinclination to expose their breasts to the eye of the accoucheur, until several or many domestic remedies have been tried and failed. In the first stage a mild astringent will arrest farther truoble; MURPHY has found Alum-whey a useful lotion; while Alum-curds may be applied as a poultice to the nipple; the infant should be applied to the breast as seldom as possible, and before doing so it is always well to cover the nipple with a circular piece of gold beater's skin, or adhesive plaster, having a hole in the centre just sufficient t leave the orifices of the milk-ducts uncovered. This will lessen the pressure and irritation of the infant's gums and render the process of nursing more tolerable. Nipple shields are generally next to useless, if not injurious. The breasts should be gently rubbled from time to time with warm oil, in order to help the milk to flow more freely and easily.

Arnica, five drops of the tincture in a wine-glass full of water, applied to the nipples several times a day, is said to be very effectual in removing the tenderness and excoriation consequent upon the first few applications of the child to the breast.

Chamomilla, may be used internally and externally in the same way as Arnica, when there is inflammatton, swelling and ulceration of the nipples.

Graphite, when there is burning, aching, cracking and tenderness of the nipples. A dose may be given every night and morning.

Sulphur, when the nipples are sore and deeply fissured; when the cracks bleed and burn.

In some severe cases Sweet-oil and Lime-water may be applied frequently; or Magnesia-ointment; or Glycerine, or Collodion; or a solution of Nitrate of Silver, in the proportion of ten grains to the ounce of water, which will form a slight eschar leaving a some cuticle after it falls off. In some of the severest and most painful cases, Morphine is the only useful external application, but it must be washed off very carefully before the child is allowed to nurse.

In order to prevent any trouble about the nipples they should be washed off gently with warm water, immediately after the child has nursed, dried carefully, and then dusted with superfine wheat-flour.

In difficult and obstinate cases Calcarea, Lycopodium, Mercurius, or Silex may be required; besides the internal use of these remedis, a fine powder of Calcarea, Lycopodium, or Silex may be applied externally; or a weak ointment of Mercurius, or a fine powder of one drachm of white oxide of Zinc to one ounce of fine powdered, or sifted arrow-root. A wash of Borax is frequently useful.

DEPRESSED NIPPLES.

According to Murphy these are extremely troublesome and render the chance of nursing almost hopeless. They may be drawn out by the breast-pump so as to enable a strong infant to seize and maintain its grasp; but more frequently if fails to do so, and the nipple gradually shrinks back to its former size and place, while the infant is moving about its mouth to seize it. Such cases as these, as well as those in which the nipples are badly formed and shaped, often oblige the practitioner to discourage the reluctant mother from making any further attempts to nurse her child. But the simple plan of Tracy (see page 21) will often prove successful; it consists in winding t bit of woollen thread or yarn two or three times around the base of 'the nipples (after this has been previously drawn out sufficiently), and tying it moderately, 'tight, but not so tight as to interfere with the free circulation of the blood. Thus, the nipple may be kept permanently and sufficiently promined; and the woollen threads may be worn constantly for many days without the least inconvenience, and with permanent good results.

If the mother still be unable to nurse her child, the secretion of milk must be lessened or prevented; the remedies for excessive secretion of milk, must be used, viz.

Aconite, if the breasts be hard and knotted, the skin hot and dry, the face red, and the patient restless and discouraged

Bryonia may be given, if the Aconite does not relieve sufficently; or *Belladonna* under nearly the same circumstances.

Calcarea is especially suitable if there be great fullness or enlargement of the breasts, with tardiness in the formation of milk.

Rhus-toxicodendron, if there is a painful distention of the breasts, with rheumatic pains throughout 'the body; swelling, heat and redness of the breasts, headache, stiffness of the joints and face. *Rhus* is very serviceable at the time of weaning.

If the patient be of a full habit of body, small doses of Stibium may be given; some milk should be drawn from the breasts at long intervals only, and a bandage or strips of adhesive plaster may be applied over them, so as to maintain a firm and equable pressure, and thus promote the absorption of the remainder. If there be much distention of the breasts, warm fomentations and warm frictions will be found very serviceable. Drinks of Citrate of Magnesia, or Cream of Tartar are said to be almost uniformly successful, when aided by low diet.

Many other affections of the breast may arise after confinement; for it must be recollected that each breast is composed of an association of small glandular masses, of in other words that each lobe is a perfect and independent gland, enjoying exclusively its own vascular and nervous system, and having its own proper duct, the separate orifice of which is at the nipple. A large quantity of interlobular cellular tissue units these lobes together, and the whole is at last surrounded by the investing fibrous membrance, or mammary fascia. Both around the margins and in front of the gland is a large quantity of fat; and there also exists much fibre-tissue in the nipple between the ducts and under the areola. Hence inflammation and its results may affect, and be limited to the nipple or areola, the cutaneous or sub-cutaneous tissue, the lobes individually or collectively, and the uniting fibro-cellular tissue; it may be either *intra*-lobular or *inter*-lobular, or both combined.—BIRKETT.

Inflammation of the minute fallicular glands scattered over the nipple, forms a peculiar variety of inflammation and fissures of the nipple. The first difficulty which the mother experiences is a sensation of heat, then of tingling or smarting with a very slight redness; the skin of the nipple becomes harsh and dry, and upon careful examination one or more small vesicles will be detected. These in time become rubbed, the skin breaks, and then a little oozing is noticed, with perhaps a minute ulcer or crack at the most painful spot. These appearances may be observed in any part of the nipple, from the apex to its base, or even upon the areola; as the mischief advances the cracks extend, taking either a circular or longitudinal course; but the former is most common. The pain now becomes very severe when the infant nurses; the fissures divide and increase in extent and depth; the skin becomes entirely destroyed, or a circular fissure surrounding the base of the nipple threatens its total destruction by sloughing. The fissures and ulcers bleed freqently so that the infant often vomits blood after nursing.

One of the most important and troublesome consequences of

this form of disease is secondary inflammation of the deep fibre-tissue uniting together the tubes or ducts in the nipple; the inflammatory exudation and induration may cause obliteration of one or more of the milk-ducts. The inflammation may also extend to the glandular tissue, and give rise to deep and numerous abscesses.

Treatment.—The preventive treatment consists in hardening the nipples as soon as quickening begins; the nipple then should be exposed to the air occasionally, washed with bland-soap and water, and wetted night and morning with a little diluted Cologne-water, or with alcohol and water, or with Arnica-water. After the birth of the child, too much care cannot be taken to see that the nipple is carefully and properly washed and cleaned after each application of the infant to the breast; the secretions from the child's mouth combined with the milk should never be suffered to become dry upon the part. The nipple should also be protected from the pressure and friction of the dress and bedclothes by some resisting body, such as a nipple-shield.

When the inflammation, fissures and abrasions are not very severe they will often yield to protection, frequent ablution, aided by some mild powder, such as Lycopodium, starch-powder, or Carbonae of Magnesia, or one drachm of White Oxide of Zinc mixed with one ounce of finely powdered and sifted arrow-root, applied after the nipple has been carefully washed and dried.

When the soreness of the nipples is produced by an aphthous inflammation of the child's mouth, a solution of Borax, or Chlorate of Potash, or the 1st dilution of Nitric-acid may be applied three or four times a day, or more.

The internal and external use of Nitrate of Silver may be tried; but the external application as ordinarily used is attended with great pain, although the second or third application is not as severe as he first.

Collodion is said to be a very useful application and preferable to most others.

Among the internal remedies, *Graphite, Sepia, Zincum*-metallicum deserve attention; also *Petroleum*, and *Sanguinaria*

MILK FEVER.

This according to Colombat is not so much a disease as a febrile movement requisite to form the secretion of milk in a woman recently delivered. It commences with shooting pains and aching in the breasts, which become swollen; the glands under the arm pit are also apt to become tender and enlarged. These symptoms generally commence on the third day after the birth of the child; in certain cases as early as the first or second and sometimes even as late as the sixth. The pulse becomes full and frequent, the skin hot and dry, face flushed, there is thirst, whitish fur on the tongue, scantiness of the urine, more or less general agitation and headache. This fever generally subsides in twenty-four hours; sometimes in the course of six, eight or twelve.

While the milk-fever lasts, the lochial discharge diminishes, or is temporarily suspended; but soon an abundant perspiration sets in, and the lochia then again become as free as before the attack.

If the child is applied early and sufficiently frequently to the breast threre is generally little or no milk-fever; the same holds true of those women who perspire very copiously.

Treatment.— If the fever runs too high and the breasts are very much swollen and painful, small doses of Aconite and Antimony should be relied upon; the breasts should also be drawn regularly, at least every four hours, and sometimes every two or three hours. The Sulphate of Potash enjoys a very long-standing repuation as an anti-lactic semedy.

ENGORGEMENT AND INFLAMMATION OF THE BREASTS.

Engorgement of the breasts generally appears on the fourth or fifth day after delivery, and principally affects persons who do not with to nurse, or who do not apply the child to be breast at least every four hours, both by night and day, or those who have too great a flow of milk and nurse a feeble child, or have

ENGORGEMENT OF THE BREASTS. 143

their nipples too small or large, or who have taken cold. The patient has chills and pain in the back followed by fever; 'the breasts become hard and unequal, but preserve their natural color; but the breasts may become coked or indurated, and the secretion of milk will then be diminished or completely suspended, while the patient has pains in the whole of 'the breast, which may even extend to the arm pits.

When *inflammation* has set in, 'the breasts gradually increase in size, and become very painful and hard; they are excessively hot and tense, and assume a reddish color; the pains lancinating and pricking; fever sets in, with headache, which increases more and more; the face is flushed, urine scanty with a whitish sediment; the fæces exhale an acid odor; and lastly the inflamed breast acquires considerable size and hardness, which may extend to the arm-pits and neck. The pains may become so acute that delirium sets in.

Simple engorgement generally terminates by resolution; while suppuration is the most common termination of the really inflammatory variety. We ascertain that suppuration is taking place by the persistence and pregressive increase of the inflammatory symptoms, and by the presence of hard lumps or cakes in the breasts, together with throbbing pains and intolerable shootings. Finally fluctuation is discovered.

Treatment.—The preventive treatment consists in applying the infant early to the breasts in order to empty them as soon as they are filled; in keeping the breasts and person of the patient warm; and by moderate diet.

When engorement has once set in, a flaxseed poultice containing a little milk, castile-soap, or ten or twelve grains of Soda, or Potash, may be applied; or Hydridate of Potash-ointment, one drachm to the ounce of simple cerate; or bits o Canton-flannel, or Spongio-piline dipped in hot Pearlash-watei not too strong.

Aconite and Antimony may be used internally; or Aconite and Bryonia; or Belladonna, or Mercurius may be given in alternation with Bellad., especially if transient chills and throbbings set in.

Phosphorus is another very useful remedy when the inflammation is active and rapid suppuration threatens; it will often be found to quickly relieve the excessive pain, redness and swelling. It is also useful against a fistulous, or indurated condition of the breast.

Hepar-sulphus is indicated after the inflammatory symptoms have somewhat abated, yet signs of suppuration are still present. It may help to produce resolution, but is also said to expedite the bursting of the abscess when it has already formed.

Nitric-acid is said to be useful, when there are hard nodosities in the breasts.

Sulphur, when there is inflammation and induration of the breasts; or erysipelatous inflammation with heat, hardness, and redness radiating from the nipple.

Lycopodium, when there are hard, burning nodosities in the breasts; with discharge of blood and sticky water from the nipples.

Conium, when there is hardness of the breasts with pains at night.

Bromine and Sabina, when there is swelling of the breasts.

Mercurius-solubilis, when there is swelling of the breasts, especially of the nipples, which are somewhat harder than natural.

Calcarea, when there is swelling and heat of the breasts, with inflammation of the nipples.

Belladonna, when there is hardness, with excessive secretion of milk, and some inflammation.

Rhus-toxicodendron, when there is painful distention of the breasts, when the milk first begins to flow, with pain and itching of the nipples.

Zincum, when there is distention of the breasts; with soreness of the nipples.

If the abscess be small, it may be allowed to open of itself but if the engorgement and induration is extensive an opening should be made as soon as fluctuation is discovered; the incision should be made in the direction of one of the radia of a circle, of which the nipples is the centre; a bit of lint or linen may be introduced into the opening to prevent its closing too soon; the fears of some homœopathic physicians about lancing abscesses are founded upon the grossest ignorance and prejudice.

ALTERATIONS OF THE MILK.

According to Colombat, after nervous diseases the milk is apt to become thin like water, or of a greenish color; it may assume a yellowish color in inflammations of the breast; a saltish and disagreeable taste in inflammatory diseases, and lastly, a sour smell after labor generally; while it contracts an odor like that of garlic in persons who eat that substance.

To discover whether the consistence of the milk is too thin, or too thick, it is merely necessary to put a drop on one of the nails; if it adheres to it at first, and then spreads without running, it is in a natural condition, if it runs; it is too thin; and if it adheres to the nail without spreading, it is too thick. In nervous women the milk is apt to be thin and not very nutritious, whilst it is also subject to important changes from the slightest vexation, or other powerful mental emotions. Menstruation renders it thin and serous; Pregnancy makes it thick and unfit for the nourishment of infants; salt-meats, highly seasoned dishes, mealy vegetables, salads and fruits make it more abundant and thinner; spirituous liquors, late hours, excessive sleep and all abundant secretions diminish it in quantity.

From the chemical examination of eighty-nine females VERNOIS and BECQUEREL have established the healthy standard of human milk, as follows:

	MEDIUM.	MAXIMUM.	MINIMUM.
Density	1032.67	1046.48	1025.61
Water	889.08	999.98	832.30
Solid constituents	110.92	147.70	83.33
Sugar	43.64	59.55	25.22
Casein and extractive matters	39.24	70.92	19.32
Butter	26.66	56.42	6.66
Salt	1.38	3.88	0.55

In twenty-six cases the influence of the presence of Colostrum from the first to the fifteenth day after delivery, was as follows:

	MAXIMUM.	MINIMUM.	MEDIUM.	MEDIUM. NORMAL STATE.
Density	1032.86	1025.61	1031.34	1032.67
Water	882.97	870.34	872.45	889.08
Solid constituents	147.70	117.03	127.55	110.92
Sugar	48.46	35.54	41.23	43.64
Casein and extractive matters	48.66	32.92	44.05	39.24
Butter	56.42	28.89	40.35	26.66
Salts	3.38	1.23	1.92	1.38

Hence the presence of colostrum causes a partial diminution of the density of milk,
constant diminution of the quantity of the water of milk.
constant increase of solid constituents,
constant but slight diminution of sugar,
notable increase of casein,
very marked increase of butter,
increase of the salts.

As regards the influence of the age of the nurse:

	15 TO 20 YEARS.	20 TO 25 YEARS.	25 TO 30 YEARS.	30 TO 35 YEARS,	35 TO 40 YEARS.	MEDIUM. NORMAL STATE.
Density	1032.24	1033.08	1032.20	1032.42	1032.74	1032.67
Water	869.85	886.91	892.96	888.06	894.94	889.08
Solids	130.15	113.09	107.04	111.94	105.06	110.92
Sugar	35.23	44.72	45.77	39.53	39.60	34.61
Casein, &c	55.74	38.73	36.53	42.33	42.07	39.24
Butter	37.38	28.21	33.48	28.61	22.33	26.66
Salts	1.90	1.43	1.26	1.44	1.06	1.38

Hence although the difference is not very great, it will be most desirable to have a wet-nurse from 20 to 30 years of age.

As regards the age of the milk, the above authors have furnished the following table:

ALTERATIONS OF THE MILK.

	1 Day to 1 Month	1 to 2 Months	2 to 3 Months	3 to 4 Months	4 to 5 Months	5 to 6 Months	6 to 7 Months	7 to 8 Months	8 to 9 Months	9 to 10 Months	10 to 11 Months	11 to 12 Months	12 to 18 Months	18 to 24 Months	Medium Normal State
Density	1031.69	1033.11	1032.70	1032.00	1032.10	1034.35	1034.97	1031.37	1032.88	1034.44	1031.61	1030.68	1034.05	1030.81	1032.67
Water	872.84	872.99	886.16	889.67	888.25	901.51	891.35	889.49	891.65	900.63	889.37	889.28	891.34	876.65	889.08
Solids	127.16	127.01	113.84	110.33	111.75	98.49	108.65	110.51	108.35	99.37	110.63	110.96	108.66	123.45	110.92
Sugar	40.40	43.13	43.37	44.47	44.66	42.00	44.18	41.52	45.31	47.62	47.06	43.91	43.92	41.33	43.64
Casein, &c.	45.38	48.26	37.92	36.96	38.28	38.63	38.86	35.02	38.79	45.84	38.57	41.06	36.98	37.32	39.24
Butter	39.55	34.05	31.22	27.59	27.31	26.57	24.35	22.79	23.06	31.06	25.03	24.61	26.44	43.47	26.66
Salts	1.83	1.59	1.33	1.31	1.50	1.29	1.26	1.18	1.19	1.28	1.22	1.38	1.32	1.33	1.38

INFLUENCE OF THE AGE OF MILK FROM 1 TO 24 MONTHS.

1. The only conclusions which can be drawn from this table are: That the milk of a nurse whose breast of milk is from 1 to 3 months old will contain *too much butter* for an infant over three months of age; and conversely; while breast-milk over 3 months old, will contain *too little butter* for a child under 3 months of age.

2. That breast-milk under 2 months old, will contain too much casein for infants over 2 months of age; and a breast of milk over 2 months of age will contain too little casein for infants under 2 months.

The quantity of sugar in breast-milk of all ages does not vary materially.

As regards the influence of the *constitution of the nurse,* it is erroneously supposed that a strong powerful wet-nurse has the best and most nourishing milk. But this is far from being the case; all her food goes to supply her own body, and hence she has but little to spare in the shape of milk.

	STRONG CONSTITUTION.	DELICATE CONSTITUTION.	MEDIUM NORMAL STATE.
Density	1032.97	1031.90	1032.67
Water	911.19	887.59	889.08
Solids	88.81	112.41	110.92
Sugar	32.55	42.88	43.64
Casein, &c.	28.98	39.21	39.24
Butter	25.96	28.78	26.66
Salts	1.32	1.54	1.38

INFLUENCE OF PREGNANCY.

	PREGNANCY FOR 3 MONTHS.	MEDIUM NORMAL STATE.
Density	1030.67	1032.67
Water	860.97	889.08
Solids	139.01	110.92
Sugar	46.47	43.64
Casein, &c.	34.52	39.24
Butter	55.97	26.66
Salts	2.05	1.38

The principal influence of pregnancy on milk is to produce a great increase in the quantity of butter; and it is remarkable that the same effect is produced in the cow, the proportion of butter increasing from 36.12 to 47.52.

THE INFLUENCE OF MENSTRUATION,

is variable; as a rule the density, quantity of water, and sugar are somewhat diminished; and that of the solids and casein decidedly increased, the butter and salt decidedly or slightly augmented. Still in two instances the solids increased from 111 and 113 to 142 and 144, and in another case, fell from 113 to 96.

The quantity of Sugar in one case fell from 54 to 35; increased in another from 39 to 47; and remained stationary at 44 in a third.

The quantity of Casein increased in one case from 35 to 40 in another from 41 to 42; and fell in a third from 41 to 39.

The quantity of Butter increased in one case from 21 to 67 in a second, from 29 to 52; and fell in a fourth, from 24 to 10.

Hence it is to be supposed that equally great changes will take place in the state of the stomach and bowels of the infant.

ALTERATIONS OF THE MILK.

INFLUENCE OF COMPLEXION AND COLOR OF THE HAIR.

It is supposed that the milk of females with brown hair is preferable to that of blondes. The milk of persons with blond hair is less dense; contains more water; less of solids, sugar, casein, and salt; and a little more of butter.

INFLUENCE OF FOOD.

In nurses who are poorly fed the quantity of water in their milk is apt to increase from 876 to 893; the solids to diminish from 123 to 104; the sugar to increase from 41 to 45; the casein to remain unaltered; and the butter to lessen from 43 to 18.

INFLUENCE OF THE QUANTITY OF THE MILK.

When the breasts furnish but little milk, the density, and water and butter are apt to increase; the solids, sugar and casein to diminish.

INFLUENCE OF ACUTE FEVERS.

	MEAN IN FEVER.	NORMAL MEAN.
Density	1031.20	1032.67
Water	884.91	889.08
Solids	115.09	110.92
Sugar	33.10	43.64
Casein, &c	50.40	39.24
Butter	29.86	26.66
Salts	1.73	1.38

Hence in fevers, there is a slight diminution of the density of the milk, and a notable lessening of the water and sugar; while there is an proportionate increase of solids, a marked augmentation of casein and butter, and a slight increase of salt.

INFLUENCE OF SEVERE MORAL EMOTION.

	MFRAL EMOTIONS.	NORMAL MEANS.
Density	1032.99	1032.67
Water	908.93	889.08
Solids	91.07	110.92
Sugar	34.92	43.64
Casein, &c	50.00	39.24
Butter	5.14	26.66
Salts	1.01	1.38

In this case there was a sudden increase of water and casein; and a very great diminution of the solids, sugar and butter.

INFLUENCE OF CHRONIC DISEASE.

	MAXIMUM.	MINIMUM.	MEDIUM.	NORMAL MEAN.
Density	1037.52	1027.07	1034.47	1032.67
Water	923.58	832.96	885.50	889.08
Solids	167.04	89.51	114.50	110.92
Sugar	51.98	30.38	43.37	43.64
Casein, &c	47.49	12.70	37.06	39.24
Butter	73.05	6.90	32.57	26.66
Salts	3.38	0.61	1.50	1.38

In acute diseases the quantity of sugar is apt to be greatly diminished; while it generally remains unaltered in chronic affections. On the other hand, the quantity of casein is frequently very much increased in acute diseases, and lessened in chronic. The density and quantity of water is lessened in both what increased. The inference would be, that when infants must acute and chronic disorders; the solids, butter, and salt some- be partly fed while their mothers are suffering from acute disease, less milk and more sugar and water should be added to their food; and more milk and less sugar in chronic affections.

INFLUENCE OF CONSUMPTION.

	Without diarrhœa, abscesses and emaciation.	With diarrhœa, &c.	Normal Mean.
Density	1031.84	1031.38	1032.67
Water	876.59	903.16	889.08
Solids	123.41	96.84	110.92
Sugar	42.14	43.45	43.64
Casein, &c	37.46	39.14	39.24
Butter	41.82	12.76	26.66
Salts	1.99	1.49	1.38

The milk of decidedly consumptive females is markedly deficient in butter.

Sugar, Casein and Butter are the principal nutrient materials in milk.

QUANTITY OF SUGAR.

	MEDIUM.	MAXIMUM.	MINIMUM.
In Health	43.64	59.55	25.22
In acute disease	33.10	48.71	19.50
In chronic disease	43.37	57.98	30.38

QUANTITY OF CASEIN.

	MEDIUM.	MAXIMUM.	MINIMUM.
In Health	39.24	70.92	193.02
In acute disease	50.40	66.26	34.62
In chronic disease	37.06	47.49	12.70

QUANTITY OF BUTTER.

	MEDIUM.	MAXIMUM.	MINIMUM.
In Health	26.66	56.42	6.66
In acute disease	29.86	56.37	5.14
In chronic disease	32.57	73.05	6.90

COMPARISON OF HUMAN AND COW'S MILK.

	MEDIUM COW'S	MEDIUM HUMANS.
Density	1033.38	1032.67
Water	864.06	889.08
Solids	135.94	110.92
Casein, &c	55.15	39.24
Sugar	38.03	43.64
Butter	36.12	26.66
Salts	6.64	1.38

Hence it is evident that cow's milk contains considerably more casein, butter and salt than human milk, and less water, and sugar. Mother's milk is always very obviously alkaline, while cow's milk is either very feebly alkaline, often neutral, and sometimes slightly acid. Therefore, when it is necessary to feed infants with cow's milk it should always be borne in mind that it was originally intended for calves and not for babies, and that it must be modified somewhat to suit the latter. In the first place more water and sugar must be added; then, as cow's milk is naturally less alkaline than mother's milk, some alkali should be added, not only to supply this deficiency but also in some measure to neutralize the effects of the excess of butter. The natural alkalies and salts, &c. of human milk are: Carbonate of Lime, Phosphate of Lime, Chloride of Sodium, Sulphate of Soda, Magnesia, Soda, Lactate of Soda, Iron, and Chloride of Potash; hence one or the other of these should be added according to the peculiarities of the constitution and other requirements of the child.

When there is an aphthous state of the mouth, with redness and dryness of the tongue and throat, a little Chlorate of Potash in the milk will prove almost specific.

When there is much acidity of the stomach, with acid vomiting, sour diarrhœa, or constipation, Calcarea, Magnesia, or Soda, may be added to the milk, according to the several indications for the use of these remedies.

When there is a general delicacy of the child with a tendency to rickets, Phosphate of Lime, or Ferrum must be used.

Alterations in the mother's milk produced by a violent fit of anger, may be corrected by Chamomilla; by grief, with Ignatia, or Aurum; by excessive jealousy, with Hyoscyamus; by taking cold, with Dulcamara.

During the time of nursing, *blood* may be discharged from the nipple, without there being crack or abrasion, or bruise about it, or the breast; this is apt to occur in some delicate women, as I have seen several remarkable instances, from local or general weakness; Kreosote, Millifolium, Argenti-nitras, and Phosphoric-acid, or Arnica are the principal remedies.

There also appear to be well authenticated cases in which milk containing *Urea* in excess has passed from the nipples in consequence of more or less derangement of the kidneys, or obstruction to the passage of urine along its natural channels. Colchicum and Nitric-acid are the best remedies.

When the milk is poor, thin and serous, altered in its quality, rather than its quantity, and unfit for the proper nourishment of the infant, Sulphur and Calcarea are the most important remedies; or Mercurius and Silex.

When the milk is yellow and bitter, Rheum; when it coagulates and curdles readily, Borax; when it is repulsive to the infant, Cin., Merc., Silex, Borax. Carbo-an., Cham., Nux., Puls., or Rheum may be required.

INCONTINENCE OF MILK.

The retentive power of the mouths of the milk-ducts on the nipple is sometimes so greatly diminished as to permit the milk when formed to flow away continually. The yellow elastic tissue forms the chief uniting medium in the nipple, and a want of it, or a loss of tone in its fibre may be the reason why incontenence occurs. The fibre tissue of the nipple differs very widely from the common uniting, or cellular tissue; even when minutely examined it presents very little ordinary cellular tissue; that of which it is formed enjoys in the highest degree, a contractile power; to the unassisted eye it has a pinkish tint, is very dense and tough in its texture; when magnified it presents the appearances peculiar to the yellow or contractile fibre. The advantage of this structure is at once clear; when the milk-ducts become distended with milk, it would quickly flow away incontinently, unless there were some arrangement to produce moderate compression upon their extremities and closure of their orifices. And this condition is found to exist particularly within a quarter of an inch of the apex the nipple, when the calibre of the ducts is small.—(BIRKETT.)

Treatment.—Borax is the most homœopathic remedy, it may be used when the milk flows from the breasts so profusely that the bed becomes wet. BIRKETT suggests that astringent lotions which are known to act so powerfully on the yellow fibre tissue may be used with advantage.

CHANGES IN THE WOMB AFTRE PARTURITION.

According to MURPHY it is necessary to have a clear apprehension of the condition of the womb after parturition from what it was before the delivery of the child.

1st, The contraction of the fibres of the womb is becoming permanent;

2d, Absorption is going forward with unusual rapidity, for in ten or twelve days the womb will be reduced to one-half or one-third of its size after delivery;

3d, The mucous surface in undergoing equally rapid changes, the residue of the ovum and after-birth is being thrown off, the ends of the large vessels which project from the surface where the after-birth was attached are again shrinking to their former size, and the tide of blood that for so many months had been flowing towards this membrane is now ebbing fast away from it;

4th, The vagina is also contracting itself with great force, and the abundant secretion which had been flowing from it is now gradually ceasing and returning to its original state.

We have, therefore, to consider under these several heads, the symptoms that present themselves while this change is going forward, especially those that require our aid in the way of treatment.—MURPHY.

AFTER-PAINS,

frequently present themselves while the womb is contracting; they are often severe, and depend upon different causes; they also occur more frequently in women who have had many children, than in those who have just given birth to their first-born.

Coagulæ collecting in the womb very commonly cause after-pains; blood is often poured slowly in the cavity of the womb, during or soon after parturition, it coagulates, distends the walls of the uterus and excites spasmodic contractions. If this happens soon after delivery the patient may experience pains as severe as labor-pains, and relief is urgently called for. In some instances this may be promptly afforded by using steady pressure over the base of the womb; the irritation excites a more powerful contraction; the clot is expelled, and the patient is relieved. This method, however can only be adopted within four or six hours after delivery; at a later period the permanent contraction of the womb cannot thus be overcome, and it is better not to make such attempts. A warm stimulant enema will excite both the action of the bowels and womb, and the same straining efforts that expel the fæces will expel the clot, and relief is

AFTER-PAINS.

experienced soon after. If not, hot fomentations and soothing applications to the abdomen will usually succeed.

Wind or flatus in the intestines also often gives rise to severe after-pains. This cause may generally be distinguished from the former by a careful examination of the abdomen; when clots are retained in the womb, the uterus is generally large, prominent and exceedingly painful on pressure; every other part of the abdomen is free from pain, and generally soft; but when *flatulence* is the cause, the abdomen is swollen and tympanitic; the womb cannot be felt, and the slightest touch gives intense pain. This very character, however, is a valuable means of distinguishing the pains so produced from those of inflammation; a slight pressure causes great pain, but if it be increased the pain diminishes until it quite disappears; if after this, the hand be suddenly withdrawn from the abdomen; the pain instantly returns with increased violence, so that MURPHY has known the patient to scream with the agony this simple act produces. When inflammation is present with the tympanitis, the greater the pressure, the greater the pain.

Treatment.—MURPHY thinks that Turpentine is the best remedy for these flatulent pains. Arnica, China, Nux, Palsatilla, Bryonia, Sulphur, Carb.-veg., Verat, and Lycopodium deserve attention.

Arnica and Bryonia are thought by some to be the best remedies for flatulent colic after delivery.

Colocynth, when there is a tightness in the upper part of the abdomen, returning at short intervals and changing into severe griping; or feeling in the whole abdomen as if squeezed between stones.

Carb.-veg., when the pain and flatulence are caused by cold, with cramping pains, distention of abdomen, and pain at short intervals.

Cocculus, when the pain is high up about the epigastrium and almost arrests the breathing, and is attended with qualmishness.

Both of these causes, viz., clots and flatulence, come into operation most frequently with women who have had many children, and for an obvious reason. The muscles of the abdomen have been so weakened by frequent pregnancies, that they give no support to the bowels, when the uterus leaves the abdomen;

consequently the intestines become over-distended with air and colic is the result; so also the womb is deprived of that equable pressure which is so important to it; it yields more readily to the distention by the clots, and in place of expelling them, allows them to accumulate and produce after-pains.

Neuralgic pains in the womb sometimes give rise to very severe suffering after confinement; the abdomen is soft and free from pain; the womb is not much increased in size, but feels unusually firm under the hand and is exceedingly painful to pressure; it is closely allied to rheumatism of the womb and dysmenorrhœa, is sometimes coupled with a chronic inflammation of the womb, which is only rendered acute when an increased flow of blood is directed towards the uterus.

Treatment.—I prefer the local application of the tincture of the Root of Aconite, over the region of the womb; from $\frac{1}{4}$ to $\frac{1}{2}$ teaspoonful may be applied every two, four, six or eight hours. Chamomilla, Pulsat., and Cocculus deserve attention; also Conium, Hyosciamus and Opium.

LOCHIAL DISCHARGE.

This flows from the womb and vagina while their mucous membranes are returning to their natural condition; at first it is bloody, because the dark grumous blood which oozes from the uterine veins is mixed with it; then it becomes greenish yellow, thick and oleaginous; and lastly thin and serous.

It may retain the *sanguineous* color too long, and this may be brighter than is safe for the patient, for then there is always risk of flooding taking place, unless she retain the horizontal position, and be kept quiet, and upon proper diet.

Treatment.—Cinnamon, Sabina, Stramonium and Secale are the principal remedies.

The thick oleaginous appearance may become *purulent,* or *muco-purulent,* and when this happens it indicates pre-existing inflammation in the vagina, or neck of the womb. The patient may recover her health so as to be able to get up and go about without much inconvenience; the discharge, however, continues and may continue for months, and is soon attended with pain in the back and loins, a sense of weight and bearing down. The persistence or increase of the discharge forms a connecting link between these symptoms and the previous confinement. Thus, the whole of her present distress will be attributed, perhaps justly, to that period. The suspicion will arise hat something happened then that should not have happened; or that something was done that should not have been done, and it is very probable that the physician will be charged with having neglected his duties, and of being the cause of all the present mischief. It is necessary to ascertain the cause of this purulent discharge, it may arise from fissures or lacerations of the neck of the womb, which have become inflamed; or there may be abrasions of the vagina, or a slough may have separated, leaving an ulcer behind; or the vagina may be generally inflammed. Any, or all of these causes will give rise to a purulent discharge, and may expose the patient to months of protracted suffering long after her delivery.

Treatment.—When there are lacerations of the neck of the womb, Aconite-, Arnica- and Calendula-waters may be used in the form of injections; ano Graphite, Mercurius-solubilis or Petroleum should be given internally.

For inflammation and ulceration of the vagina, Ammon.-carb., Ambrá-grisia, Cantharides, Mercurius-solubilis, Nitric-acid, Secale, Sulphur, or Thuja, may be tried.

Calcarea may be given when the discharge continues long, without being profuse, but weakens the patient and deranges her digestive organs; also when the flow is mucous, watery and abundant, attended with much flatulence, pains, difficult digestion, diarrhœa and deficient secretion of milk.

Pulsatilla, when the discharge is thick and mucous, with pains in the loins, and despondency.

Sepia, if it is liquid and serous, or acrid and excoriating, or purulent, with induration or ulceration of the neck of the womb.

Mercurius, when the discharge is most abundant at night, and there is a tendency to inflammation of the abdominal, or sexual organs.

Sulphur, when the discharge enfeebles the woman, and does not yield to the other remedies; also Secale.

Sepia and Kreosote are also useful when the lochia are fetid, or insupportably putrid; injections of a solution of Chlorate of

Potash, or of Chloride of Zinc, or of Nitrate of Lead may be used.

SUPPRESSION OF THE LOCHIA.

Warm and moist applications should be applied to the vulva.

Aconite is indicated when the suppression occurs soon after delivery, and the patient has pains or inflammation in the abdomen, with anxiety, fever, and congestion to the chest or head. The tincture of the Root of Aconite should be applied freely over the region of the womb, if inflammation sets in.

Chamomilla, when the suppression is secondary to diarrhœa, colics, or nervous distress in the head or teeth; a cup of warm Chamomilla-tea may be allowed from time to time.

Bryonia is useful when the lochia are suppressed, attended with headache, fulness and heaviness of the head, backache, or severe stitch in the side with cough, with or without scanty secretion of hot urine.

Colocynth, when the check is accompanied by violent colics, with great flatulence and tympanitic swelling of the abdomen, with or without diarrhœa.

Pulsatilla, if the milk be also much diminished or suppressed.

Belladonna, Stramonium or Hyosciamus if there are violent pains in the head, redness of the face, dilatation of the pupils frightful dreams, or delirium.

Platina, Secale and Nux, when the lochia are scanty and offensive.

POST-PARTEM INFLAMMATION.

Inflammation of the womb and its appendages is a frequent consequence of parturition; the passages are left in a such a condition that a very slight cause may light up inflammation; the form which this assumes is as various as the causes which produce it. The inflammation may be confined to the vagina and mucous membrane of the womb; it may involve the substance and body of the womb, ovaries, or peritonæum; or the veins of the womb may be its seat. It may be acute, or sub-acute, sthenic or phlegmonous, or asthenic and typhoid.—(MURPHY.)

INFLAMMATIONS OF THE MUCOUS MEMBRANE OF THE VAGINA WOMB.

This form is generally met with after a severe labor with the first child; the vagina is less disposed to yield to the pressure and distention to which it is exposed, hence congestion arises and inflammation may follow; too frequent vaginal examinations may be exciting cause.

The *symptoms* are chiefly local; the patient complains of a great degree of soreness at the vulva; the urine is retained, which is perhaps the first symptom which attracts attention the lochial discharge is more than usually offensive; and the patient is wakeful and restless. *Retention of urine* is the most important complication, and if an attempt is made to pass the catheter, the pain is excruciating if it should not pass at once into the urethra, for the vulva being inflamed, the nymphæ, vestibule, orifice of the urethra, and especially the clitoris, are all exceedingly tender; the trumpet-shaped opening of the urethra is altogether changed, leaving only a pin-hole opening, which is not easily discovered.

The pulse is generally frequent and hard; the abdomen may be perfectly free from tenderness; the womb may bear pressure without inconvenience; the iliac region and groins may be without pain, but this frequent pulse is a certain index that there is irritation or inflammation somewhere, and the probability is that it has its seat in the mucous membrane of the vagina.

Simple inflammation of the vagina may terminate in resolution without any injury abrasion of the passages; or it may be followed by abrasions and superficial ulcerations of the mucous membranes; or it may end in slough. The last is the only serious result, because the seat of the slough is usually so unfavorable; the urethra from the pressure of the head against the pubis, is sometimes so bruised, that a slough is the result, and fistula the consequence; hence may be established one of the most unmanageable and distressing affections to which the parturient female can be exposed, viz, a constant dribbling of urine through the vagina. Other sloughs may affect the womb, vagins, or the retriculate cellular tissue between them and the peritonæum, giving rise to lacerations of the womb, disease of the neck, or those extensive suppurations that are described as pelvic abscesses; or peritonitis may result.

Treatment.—Warm emollient vaginal injections of flaxseed, slippery elm, quince-seeds, or marsh-mallow, or decoction of poppies, or warm fomentations and ablutions of the vulva may be used.

Aconite and Stibium should be given internally; or Pulsatilla, Copaiba, and other remedies for inflammation of the vagina.

Asthenic inflammation of the vagina is a far more serious result of labor, for the whole vagina is often quickly engaged in the inflammation which sometimes extends to the womb; it tendency is to rapid gangrene, which is not confined to a small space, but soon extends over a large surface, forming extensive sloughs.

The *symptoms* are: the dark, foul and offensive lochia; a certain amount of tenderness and soreness of the valva and vagina; while the attending typhoid or irritative fever is very characteristic. The rapid pulse, dry furred tongue, burning surface and sallow aspect, are the common characters of this fever, whether the cause be in the vagina, or in the womb; but MURPHY has observed that when the vagina is thus inflamed, pimples appear about the lips, which soon become pustules that form dark crusts, and thus, besides the usual sordes about the teeth and gums, the mouth is sometimes encircled by a chain of these pustules in different stages of maturity. There may be erysipelatous inflammation of the vagina, without true puerperal fever.

Treatment.—Antiseptic injections should be used, such as the solutions of Chloride of Soda, or Chlorate of Potash, or Kreosote-water, &c. Arsenicum is the most important internal remedy and should be given frequently and freely, assisted or not by China and Camphor.

If sloughing take place, great attention must be paid to the manner in which the denuded surfaces heal, lest adhesions, or great contractions of the vagina take place; a small cylindrical bougie should be carefully passed daily as far as the os-uteri, and the surfaces touched lightly with a weak solution of Nitric acid, or Nitrate of Silver.

INFLAMMATION OF THE CAVITY OF THE NECK OF THE WOMB.

This is generally of a chronic character, and may be recognized by the appearance of a viscid mucous discharge, either mixed with the lochia, or continuing long after their decline. It may be the result of lacerations of the neck of the womb, or only of the mucous membrane that lines it.

The *symptoms* are seldom so severe as to interfere much with the patient's recovery; she is generally able to get up and go about at the usual time, only she complains of a dull aching pain about the loins and over the small of the back, increased by the upright position and by exercise, but relieved by rest; she also speaks of a whitish viscid mucus passing from the vagina.

Treatment.—This generally cannot well be undertaken until the lochial discharge has ceased, and the viscid mucus alone remains. Graphite may be given internally, or Nitric-acid; while a solution of Nitrate of silver may be applied to the surface every fourth or sixth day.

Inflammation of the mucous membrane of the cavity of the womb seldom occurs alone; either the fibrous structure of the womb becomes engaged, or the inflammation extends to the uterine veins.

INFLAMMATION OF THE FIBROUS STRUCTURE OF THE WOMB.

Is generally the result of a severe and protracted labor, or of sudden exposure to cold air, cold applications to the womb, or from allowing the woman to lie too long in her wet clothes.

The *symptoms* generally appear in about forty-eight hours after delivery; the pulse continues frequent, about one hundred, and full; there is tenderness on pressure, either in the right or left groin, more generally the left; the body of the womb feels rather larger and firmer than usual, but if slightly touched the patient does not complain, although if it be firmly compressed, the pain produced will be very great; the lochial discharge is apt to be suppressed, and the milk may not be secreted. If the inflammation be not promptly subdued, chills, thirst and symptomatic fever will set in, and the inflammation seldom remains stationary, but soon extends to the neighboring tissues, especially the peri-

K

tonæum, when the nature of the case is completely altered, and danger to the patient much increased.

Treatment.—This should be prompt; tenderness over the womb or groins, attended with fever and quick pulse, should be met by the free and frequent application of the tincture of the Root of Aconite, over the whole hypogastric region. Aconite, Stibium, Bryonia, Mercurius, &c. may be given internally. Warm fomentations may be applied to the region of the womb, and to the vulva.

INFLAMMATION OF THE PERITONÆUM.

This is generally a consequence of preceeding inflammation of the fibrous tissue of the womb; metro-peritonitis is, perhaps, the most frequent form of inflammation we meet with after labor. It may be partial and confined to the immediate neighborhood of the womb, or general and spread over the whole peritoneum. (MURPHY.)

The *symptoms* are sufficiently distinct. Locally, the tenderness of the womb, and in either groin, is greater than in simple metritis; *slight* pressure causes much pain, which becomes intolerable if the pressure be increased. That portion of the abdomen about the seat of the inflammation becomes swollen and puffy, so as to render the outline of the womb undefined. The pulse is quick, wiry and incompressible; the countenance anxious; the tongue rather dry, with red edges and tip; there is nausea and sometimes vomiting.

If the inflammation be not at once subdued, it will spread rapidly over the whole abdomen, the swelling of which becomes general, accompanied by great tenderness over the entire surface; the pulse becomes still more contracted and wiry, and the countenance more expressive of intense suffering. Vomiting now becomes incessant, the respirations labored, and any effort at respiration very painful and distressing, as the motions of the diaphragm, &c., disturb the necessary quiet of the inflamed parts; hence the patient lies on her back, having her knees drawn up and her chest raised, so as to prevent as much as possible the pain that inspiration produce; her breathing is never full and deep, but each breath is cut short by a rapid expiration, sometimes accompanied by a cough. The bowels are constipated, and the skin dry, with the exception of irregular partial sweat about the neck.

These acute symptoms rarely continue beyond twelve or twenty-four hours, for if the inflammation is not soon controlled, they are succeeded by those of constitutional exhaustion. The abdomen becomes perfectly tympanitic, but sometimes loses its acute tenderness; the pulse becomes extremely rapid, one hundred and fifty or one hundred and sixty, and feeble; the countenance cadaverous; the vomiting no longer continues convulsive, but a greenish fluid is ejected from the stomach, with little or no effort; violent diarrhœa sets in; the extremities become cold, and the surface more or less covered with a greasy perspiration; such symptoms soon prove fatal.

Treatment.—MURPHY decides that the ordinary allopathic treatment of free depletion, followed by purgatives and mercury, is very questionable in propriety; excessive depletion hastens and confirms the stage of constitutional exhaustion, while Mercury is apt to cause an exhausting and fatal diarrhœa as soon as the inflammation subsides, and purgatives are positively injurious, because by exciting the peristaltic of the bowels, newly formed adhesions are disturbed, and the inflammation is renewed; nature endeavors, he says, to guard against these accidents by the supervention of an obstinate constipation, which often resists even active purgatives. So long as the neighboring tissue the peritonæum is actively inflamed, the mucous membrane is torpid, but as soon as the peritonitis yields the mucous membrane becomes involved, as is manifest by the diarrhœa that follows.

In opposition to this stereotype and ruinous treatment, MURPHY is inclined to recommend the free use of Opium; it not only allays the high degree of nervous irritation, but also exerts a direct antiphlogistic effect.

Fomentations, hot bran, or flaxseed poultices may be applied to the abdomen; but the most important part of the external treatment, is the free and frequent application of the tincture of the Root of Aconite, viz, from a half to a whole teaspoonful, every two, four or six hours, according to the severity of the symptoms.

I claim the credit of being the first to point out the really homœopathic remedies of peritonitis, (see Homœopathic Examiner, Vol. I. New Series, p. 338). The Mineral-acids, Colocynth, and Mercurius-corrosivus, are the only true homœopathic remedies. According to CHRISTISON, in poisoning with the Mineral-acids, the outer or peritoneal surface of the abdominal viscera is *commonly* either very vascular, or bears even more unequivocal signs of inflammation, viz, effusion of fibrin, or adhesions among the different turns of the intestines. In this respect, the action of the Mineral-acids differs from that of most metallic remedies, which, with the exception of Mercurius-corrosivus, very seldom cause unequivocal peritoneal inflammation. It is singular, for instance, that however severe the inflammation of the mucous membrane of the stomach and bowels caused by Arsenicum may be, inflammatory redness of the peritoneal coat is seldom or never found; this contrasts strongly with the almost specific of the Mineral-acids, Mercurius-corrosivus and Colocynth in causing *bona fide* peritonitis.

Colocynth is said to be of great service, even in desperate cases, when the abdomen is greatly distended and the pains insupportable, so that the patient cannot bear the least motion, or pressure from the bed-clothes, but lies with her thighs drawn up to the abdomen as closely as possible; also when there is diarrhœa with colicky pains every time the patient drinks.

Mercurius-solubilis and *corrosivus* are best suited against the early and acutely inflammatory stage, or when there are signs of effusion in the peritonæum; when the patient has a dejected and apprehensive look, with burning and almost inextinguishable thirst, flow of saliva, burning and cutting pains in the abdomen, with straining and bearing down to stool, with mucous and bloody discharges; high colored and offensive urine, general and debilitating sweats.

Nitric, or *Muriatic*-acid is indicated, when the stage of exhaustion has commenced to set in.

Bryonia is probably more indicated against rheumatic inflammation of the womb, than in true peritonitis; still its well known efficacy in pleurisy speaks somewhat for its application in the treatment of inflammations of other serous membranes.

Chamomilla is doubtless not at all homœopathic to peritonitis, but surely to pain and flatulent distention of the abdomen.

Nux, Rhus, Arsenicum, Hyoscyamus, Stramonium, Platina and other remedies are probably only homœopathic to some of the symptoms or accidents of peritonitis, than to the disease itself.

INFLAMMATION OF THE SUB-PERITONEAL TISSUE.

This is usually observed at a later period after delivery, than the preceding inflammations; it may occur about the twelfth or fourteenth day and often arises from the extention of a previously existing inflammation of the womb; hitherto this variety of puerperal disease has been but little understood; it was only when it terminated in the formation of extensive abscesses that it received any attention.

The *symptoms* which characterise it are frequently disguised by the more prominent symptoms of the antecedent inflammation; thus an attack of metritis may seem to yield, the womb becomes free from pain on pressure, the abdomen is soft, and the patient only complains of inability to move which she attributes to weakness rather than pain; but the pulse remains frequent, and a slight chill may have taken place. If these signs pass unnoticed, the increasing weakness of the patient chiefly attracts attention; the chills may return, followed by irregular perspirations; she sleeps badly, and may complain of pain in passing water or fæces; sometimes a diarrhœa sets in. If the lochial discharge has not subsided, it becomes very much diminished, and the breasts shrink considerably; one or the other leg often becomes the seat of severe neuralgic pains, and finally is found to be swollen and œdematous, as well as retracted, or drawn up to the body. If there be no fixed pain at any part of the abdomen, or groin, still a careful examination will detect some swelling, hardness or resistance. Finally, if the abscess be seated in the iliac fossa it will point in one or the other groin; abscess within the sheath of the iliacus internus and psoas muscles generally works its way down to the upper and inner part of the thigh, or more rarely it points in the lumbar region. Pus in the broad ligaments, or any other of the intra-pelvic folds of the peritonæum, will in all probability burst either into the womb, or vagina, bladder or rectum, or into the cavity of the peritonæum. When there is much irritation of the bladder or rectum, or difficulty in passing water, or fæces, careful rectal and vaginal examinations should be frequently made in order to detect and let out the matter as soon as possible; it is not only allowable, but decidedly desirable to puncture the rectum or vagina in order to empty the abscess as early as possible.

Treatment.—The local application of Aconite over the whole hypogastrium, and repeated every two, four or six hours; Aconite and Stibium internally.

At a very early period the peculiar treatment of suppurative inflammation must be put in force. Tartar-emetic and Hepar-sulphur are peculiarily homœopathic to suppuration.

There are a variety of theories about the formation of pus; one is, that the pus globules are blood globules deprived of their colored envelopes, altered, swollen and enlarged. Another, is that it arises from an alteration of the plastic or inflammatory lymph, or from the buffy coat of inflamed blood, which is thus skimmed off. PAGET says that the most frequent degeneration of inflammatory lymph is into pus, and that many of the varieties of pus owe their peculiarities to the coincident degenerations of the fibrin effused in inflammations; thus, if we watch the process of an abscess, we may find one day a circumscribed, hard, and quite solid mass of coagulable lymph or fibrine, and in a few days later the solid mass has become fluid; now the solidity and hardness are due to inflammatory lymph; the later fluid is pus, and the change is the conversion of lymph into pus. It is generally said that suppurative inflammation has then taken place in the centre of the swelling, and that its effects are bounded by the plastic or adhesive inflammation; it might be said with greater justice, that of a certain quantity of lymph deposited in the original area of inflammation, the central portions have degenerated into pus, while the outer portions have been maintained, or even have become more highly developed.

A third theory is that pus arises from a solution of the fat contained in the inflamed part, and in proof, it has been found that pus contains from twenty-three to twenty-six, or twenty-eight parts in a thousand of fat and cholesterine, while mucus contains only two or three parts. The serum of pus also contains from twelve to thirteen thousandths of chloride of Sodium, while that of the blood contains only ferom four to five.

Staphysagria is said to be specific against inflammatory suppurations; *Plumbum-aceticum* is said to cause the suppurative process to cease. Sulphur, Silex, Kali-hydriod., and Mercurius are thought to be homœopathic to different varieties of suppuration.

If these means fail to arrest the progress of the suppuration, if chills take place, if the vagina become fuller, the womb more fixed and other evidences of the formation of a large quantity of pus be present, it will be necessary to support the strength of the patient, because the quantity of pus which accumulates is in almost direct proportion to her weakness. China, Wine and Opium, with a nutritious diet, are then essential.

INFLAMMATION OF THE VEINS OF THE WOMB.

This may be the consequence of a severe labor; it sometimes follows violent floodings, as the cold applications so often used may excite violent reaction and inflammation of these veins; the removal of an adherent placenta also predisposes to it; or it may arise from the absorption of putrid matter from the fragments of a retained placenta, &c.

The *symptoms* are of a typhoid character; a chill occurs when the milk should appear, no secretion of milk takes place, the pulse becomes rapid and unsteady, the tongue dry, the face pinched and sallow, the skin hot, without perspiration, the patient is restless, sleepless and sometimes incoherent; the lochial discharge is very offensive. As the inflammation proceeds, the chills return at irregular intervals; the pulse increases in frequency; the tongue becomes furred; sordes form about the teeth; the face becomes more sallow and shrunk; the eye glassy; muttering delirium sets in; the whole surface is yellow and burning; petichiæ and profuse sweats sometimes burst out.

The patient may die in two or three days; but if the patient is to recover some distant part becomes inflamed and the uterine phlebitis subsides; thus, the armpit, leg, groin or buttock may become the seat of an inflammation which usually terminates in the formation of pus, and when it is discharged the patient soon recovers.

Treatment.—There is no form of inflammation that prostrates the vital powers more completely than this; the treatment should therefore be chiefly stimulant; weak solutions of Chlorate of Soda or Potash may be injected into the vagina to correct the fetor of the discharge; and China, Arsenicum, Kreosote, or Secale should be given freely

ADHESIVE INFLAMMATION OF THE CRURAL AND PELVIC VEINS.
(Milk-Leg).

This is a sub-acute, or chronic, or more properly, a plastic inflammation of the veins in connexion with the womb; it may begin on the twelfth day after delivery, and sometimes as late as the twentieth.

The *symptoms* are: a chill more or less distinct, some headache and nausea, quick small pulse, irritability and anxiety; the patient then soon complains of pain and uneasiness about the pelvis; she is restless, but cannot move without pain; she describes it as extending from the groin down the thigh and leg, or perhaps she may be seized with a violent cramp-like pain in the calf of the leg, or in the muscles of the hip; the groin in soon discovered to be tumid, and the swelling extends down the thigh and leg, so that in a day or two the whole limb is greatly enlarged, tense, shining and elastic; the pain then diminishes, but the limb is immoveable. In some instances the swelling begins from below, in the ham, or calf of the leg, or ankle, and extends upwards. Pain is soon excited if the lymphatic glands or venous trunks are passed upon; red lines or spots may be observed along the course of the lymphatics; the veins feel hard and knotted like whip-cord. The pulse often rises to one hundred and forty, small, quick and weak; the tongue is white, face, pillid there is thirst and some nausesa the lochia and milk are gererally arrested. The patient give very little sleep, and is often bathed in the morning in a profuse perspiration.

This stage of the attack often lasts ten or fourteen days, when the patient gradually begins or recover, but she may remain lame even for months after the attack.

Treatment.—The tincture of the Root of Aconite should be applied freely over the course of the inflamed veins and lymphatics; Aconite should also be given internally.

Belladonna will relieve the crampy pain in the calf of the leg, together with the swelling and inflammation of the veins and lymphatics, especially if there is a teaching pain in the leg, rending in the joints, and a red blush over the limb.

Bryonia is most useful in the chronic stage, after the use of Aconite, Stibium, or Belladonna; especially when there are darwing and shooting pains from the hips to the feet; general perspiration; great tenderness of the leg to touch or motion; pain in the back, loins, hips and lower part of the abdomen; stiffness and swelling without redness.

Pulsatilla is most indicated when the veins are more involved than the lymphatics.

Rhus, when there is a chronic swelling, with great weakness of the leg, and a typhoid condition.

Arsenicum, when the patient is very low, typhoid or hectic, with delirium, or melancholy with excessive anguish, with severe burning nocturnal pains, in the tumid and œdematous limb.

China, when the same symptoms are present and the attack has come on after profuse flooding.

Mercurius, Sulphur and Antimony when suppuration threatens to set in.

Calcarea and Iodine when the patient is scrofulous.

Sepia, when there is chronic congestion inflanation of the womb.

PUERPERAL MANIA.

will be fully treated of in a forthcomng work on Nervous diseases and Mental derangements.

EXCESSIVE LACTATION.

Many poor women nurse their children from eighteen months to two years in the belief that they will thus prevent pregnancy; some delicate women who have had two or three children in quick succession may have all the symptoms arising from undue suckling, when her infant is not more than two or three months old.

Symptoms.—The earliest symptoms is a dragging sensation in the back when the child is in the act of nursing, and an exhausted feeling of sinking and emptiness afterwards; soon followed by loss of appetite, costiveness and pain in the left side, then the head becomes affected almost with giddiness, great depression of spirits, sometimes with much throbbing and singing in the ears. Dry cough, short breathing and palpitation may come on from the slightest exertion. Finally the patient becomes pale, thin and weak; night-sweats, swelling of the ankles, and nervousness ensue.

Treatment.—Weaning should be commenced early; the attempt to force the supply of milk by large and frequent quantities of beer, wine or spirits will only tend to the more perfect exhaustion of the mother. If cocoa, wine-whey, weak milk, punch, caudle, milk and water, cheese, &c. aided by frictions of the breasts, do not suffice to keep up the strength of the patient and a full supply of good milk, all farther attempts should at once be abandoned.

China is the most important remedy when there is much weakness, noises in the ears, palpitation of the heart, swelling of the legs, &c., especially if the patient has been subject to night-sweats, flowing, or leucorrhœa.

Causticum when the patient is irritable and easily vexed; vehement, or obstinately opiniated; forgetful, nervous, anxious or despondent; with headache, noises in the ears, dimness of sight; great appetite followed by emptiness and sense of goneness soon after eating, twitchings and jerkings in various parts of the body.

Calcarea and *Phosphorus* when the patient is scrofulous, chlorotic or inclined to consumption, &c.

Lycopodium, Pulsatilla, Rhus and Bryonia are often useful.

WEANING.

The average period for partial weaning, at least, is about the ninth month. When weaning is decided upon the mother should remain quiet for several days, or at least use her arms but very little; take light nourishment; drink as little as possible, and keep the breasts warm. The kidney and bowels should be gently acted upon, not only to aid in diminishing or dispersing the milk, but also to prevent that depression of spirits, lassitude, loss of appetite, and general derangement of the health which so frequently follow weaning when these medicines have been omitted.

Bryonia may be given if the milk continue in excessive quantity.

Belladonna, if there be much redness and painful distention of the breasts.

Pulsatilla, Rhus and Calcarea are important remedies. VAN SWIETEN has known the flow of milk to yield when an ounce or two of a strong infusion of *Sage* was taken every three hours. *Phosphoric*-acid is supposed to have a specific effect in carrying off the milk through the kidneys. Frictions of the breast with warm sweet oil, or Camphor, or Hartshorn, or Opium liniment are said to be useful.

The management of infants from their birth upwards is given so fully in Hartmann's Diseases of Children, translated by Dr. Hempel, that it is superfluous to treat of it here.

APPENDIX.

It has been thought that the value of this work would be increased by adding in the form of an Appendix, the substance of a book, by Dr. A. F. A. Desberget, of Erfurt, which has been translated from the German, under the title of the "LADIES' PERPETUAL CALANDAR. The translator remarks in relation to it, that "its utility must be at once apparent to every lady who favors it with her inspection. In Germany, its popularity is very considerable, as it tenders the service of a faithful and confidential friend, especially to the young and newly married, in matters of urgent interest,—where the inexperienced might hesitate, or not even know how to go about to ask advice."

"The manner of reckoning with reference to the time of expected confinement, is a subject which the sex,—particularly the junior members of it,—ought clearly to understand. Much time is saved, and often great anxiety avoided, by being able confidently to approximate to the hour of solicitude and hope. In point of economy, too, it is submitted, that the advantage of bespeaking the assistance of the medical and other attenddants at the proper time, is not to be overlooked: while to the latter parties, neither is it of little consequence that they are not kept in suspense,—perhaps suffering serious disappointment,—owing to the miscalculations of their patient.

The most valuable part of this book is the calendar, which is used as follows: The regular period of pregnancy,—or the time from conception till confinement,—is ten lunar months, or forty weeks, which amount to 280 days. It is frequently calculated at nine calendar months, that is to say, 273 days, or thirty-nine weeks: but we have reason to consider forty weeks as the after reckoning. When the date of conception is known, the reckoning begins from that day. If the time of conception be not known, then the reckoning must commence from the day of the last monthly appearance. Look for this date in the first column of the following tables, under the proper month, and the corresponding dates of the middle and end of pregnancy will be found standing in the same line.

If neither the day of conception be known, nor the period of the last appearance be recollected,—then, the time of *quickening,* or when the first motions of the child were perceived, must be made use of. Finding this date in the middle column of the table, the respective dates of the beginning and end of pregnancy will be found to correspond. Thus, suppose the day of quickening to be the 14th of March: look for the table in which March stands in the *middle* column, (the October table), and it will be seen that the confinement may be expected on the 2nd of August. We give the various saints' days and holydays in the calendar, because it is the custom with many women to reckon from dates of that description. The moveable feasts, however, such as Easter, Whitsuntide, &c., are omitted, as less suited for the purpose. By the "Begining," in the following tables, we mean the time of *conception* by the "Middle", the period of *quickening,* and by the "End," the time of *labor.*

JANUARY.

BEGINNING.	MIDDLE.	END.
JANUARY	MAY.	OCTOBER.
1 Circumcision	20 Frances	8 Ephraim
2 Abel	21 Prudens	9 Denys
3 Enoch	22 Helena	10 Amelia
4 Titus	23 Desiderius	11 Burkard
5 Simeon	24 Esther	12 Erenfried
6 Epiphany	25 Urban	13 Edward Conf.
7 Melchior	26 Augustine	14 William
8 Lucian	27 Bede	15 Hedwig
9 Caspar	28 William	16 Gallus
10 Paul Hermit	29 Maximilian	17 Etheldreda
11 Erhard	30 Wigan	18 Luke
12 Reynold	31 Petronella	19 Ptolemy
	JUNE.	
13 Hilarius	1 Nicomede	20 Wendelia
14 Felix	2 Macarius	21 Ursula
15 Habakkuk	3 Erasmus	22 Corduca
16 Marcellus	4 Ulrica	23 Severus
17 Anthony	5 Boniface	24 Solomon
18 Prisca	6 Benignus	25 Crispin
19 Ferdinand	7 Lucretia	26 Amandus
20 Fabian	8 Medard	27 Sabina
21 Agnes	9 Barnimus	28 Simon and Jude
22 Vincent	10 Onuphrius	29 Engelard
23 Emerantia	11 Barnabas	30 Hartman
24 Timothy	12 Blandina	31 Wolfgang
		NOVEMBER.
25 Paul	13 Tobias	1 All Saints
26 Polycarp	14 Modestus	2 All Souls
27 Chrysostom	15 Vitus	3 Gotlieb
28 Charles	16 Justina	4 Charlotte
29 Samuel	17 Alban	5 Eric
30 Adelgunda	18 Paulina	6 Leonard
31 Valerius	19 Gervase	7 Erdman

FEBRUARY.

BEGINNING.	MIDDLE.	END.
FEBRUARY.	JUNE.	NOVEMBER.
1 Bridget	20 Edward	8 Claude
2 Purific. of Mary	21 Jacobina	9 Theodore
3 Blaise	22 Acharius	10 Jonas
4 Veronica	23 Basilius	11 Martin
5 Agatha	24 JOHN BAPTIST	12 Cunibert
6 Dorothea	25 Elogius	13 Britius
7 Richard	26 Jeremias	14 Lewin
8 Solomon	27 Seven Sleepers	15 Machutus
9 Apollonia	28 Leo	16 Ottoman
10 Renata	29 PETER and PAUL	17 Hugh
11 Euphrosyne	30 Paul	18 Gotschalk
	JULY.	
12 Severinus	1 Theobald	19 Elizabeth
13 Benigna	2 Visita. of Mary	20 Edmund
14 Valentine	3 Cornelius	21 Presentation
15 Formosus	4 Martin	22 Cecilia
16 Juliana	5 Anselm	23 Clement
17 Constantia	6 Isaiah	24 Lebrecht
18 Concordia	7 Thom. a Becket	25 Catharine
19 Susanna	8 Kilian	26 Conrade
20 Euchariu	9 Cyril	27 Lot
21 Eleanor	10 Felicity	28 Gunter
22 Peter	11 Pius	29 Noah
23 Reynard	12 Henry	30 ANDREW
		DECEMBER
24 MATTHIAS	13 Margaret	1 Arnold
25 Victor	14 Bonaventure	2 Candida
26 Nestor	15 Swithin	3 Cassian
27 Hector	16 Eustace	4 Barbara
28 Justus	17 Alexis	5 Abigail

MARCH.

BEGINNING.	MIDDLE.	END.
MARCH.	JULY.	DECEMBER.
1 Albin	18 Caroline	6 Nicholas
2 Louisa	19 Ruth	7 Antonia
3 Cunigund	20 Elias	8 Conception
4 Adrian	21 Daniel	9 Joachim
5 Frederick	22 Magdalen	10 Judith
6 Everard	23 Albertine	11 Waldemar
7 Perpetua	24 Christine	12 Epimachus
8 Philemon	25 JAMES	13 Lucy
9 Prudentius	26 Anne	14 Israel
10 Henrietta	27 Berthold	15 Johanna
11 Rosina	28 Innocent	16 Ananias
12 Gregory, M.	29 Martha	17 Lazarus
13 Ernest	30 Beatrice	18 Christopher
14 Zacchary	31 Germain	19 Manasses
	AUGUST.	
15 Isabella	1 Peter	20 Abraham
16 Syriac	2 Gustavus	21 THOMAS
17 Patrick	3 Augustus	22 Beata
18 Edward	4 Perpetua	23 Ignatius
19 Joseph	5 Dominick	24 Adam and Eve
20 Rupert	6 Transfiguration	25 CHRIST BORN
21 Benedict	7 Donatus	26 STEPHEN
22 Casimer	8 Ladislaus	27 JOHN
23 Everard	9 Romanus	28 INNOCENTS
24 Gabriel	10 Lawrence	29 Jonathan
25 Annunciation	11 Titus	30 David
26 Emanuel	12 Clara	31 Sylvester
		JANUARY.
27 Hubert	13 Hildebrand	1 CIRCUMCISION
28 Gideon	14 Eusebius	2 Abel
29 Eustace	15 Assumption	3 Enoch
30 Guido	16 Isaac	4 Titus
31 Philip	17 Bertram	5 Simeon

APRIL.

BEGINNING.	MIDDLE.	END.
APRIL.	AUGUST.	JANUARY.
1 Theodore	18 Emilia	6 EPIPHANY
2 Theodosia	19 Sebald	7 Melchior
3 Christian	20 Bernard	8 Lucian
4 Ambrose	21 Athanasius	9 Caspar
5 Maximus	22 Oswald	10 Paul Hermit
6 Sixtus	23 Zaccheus	11 Erhard
7 Celestine	24 BARTHOLOMEW	12 Reynold
8 Heilman	25 Lewis	13 Hilarius
9 Bogislaus	26 Irenæus	14 Felix
10 Ezekiel	27 Gebard	15 Habakkuk
11 Herman	28 Augustine	16 Marcellus
12 Julius	29 John	17 Anthony
13 Justin	30 Benjamin	18 Prisca
14 Tiburtius	31 Rebecca	19 Ferdinand
	SEPTEMBER.	
15 Obadiah	1 Giles	20 Fabian
16 Cariseus	2 Rachel	21 Agnes
17 Rodolph	3 Mansuetus	22 Vincent
18 Florence	4 Moses	23 Emerantia
19 Werner	5 Nathaniel	24 Timothy
20 Sulpitius	6 Magnus	25 PAUL
21 Adolphus	7 Enurchus	26 Polycarp
22 Lothario	8 Mary	27 Chrysostom
23 GEORGE	9 Bruno	28 Charles
24 Albert	10 Sosthenes	29 Samuel
25 MARK	11 Gerard	30 Adelgunda
26 Raymar	12 Otilia	31 Valerius
		FEBRUARY.
27 Anastasius	13 Christlieb	1 Bridget
28 Theresa	14 Exaltation	2 Purific. of Mary
29 Sibylla	15 Constantia	3 Blaise
30 Joshua	16 Euphemia	4 Veronica

MAY.

BEGINNING.	MIDDLE.	END.
MAY.	**SEPTEMBER.**	**FEBRUARY.**
1 Philip & James	17 Lambert	5 Agatha
2 Sigismund	18 Sigfred	6 Dorothea
3 Holy Cross	19 Januarius	7 Richard
4 Florian	20 Frederica	8 Solomon
5 Gothard	21 Matthew	9 Apollonia
6 John Evangelist	22 Maurice	10 Renata
7 Godfrey	23 Joel	11 Euphrosyn
8 Stanislaus	24 John	12 Severinus
9 Job	25 Cleophas	13 Benigna
10 Gordian	26 Cyprian	14 Valentine
11 Mamertus	27 Cosmo	15 Formosus
12 Pancratius	28 Wenzel	16 Juliana
13 Servatius	29 Michael	17 Constantia
14 Christiana	30 Jerome	18 Concordia
	OCTOBER.	
15 Sophia	1 Remigius	19 Susanna
16 Honoratus	2 Volrade	20 Eucharius
17 Pascal	3 Ewald	21 Eleanor
18 Livorius	4 Francis	22 Peter
19 Dunstan	5 Charity	23 Reynard
20 Frances	6 Faith	24 Matthias
21 Prudens	7 Hope	25 Victor
22 Helena	8 Ephraim	26 Nestor
23 Desiderius	9 Denys	27 Hector
24 Esther	10 Amelia	28 Justus
		MARCH.
25 Urban	11 Burkard	1 Albin
26 Augustine	12 Erenfried	2 Louisa
27 Bede	13 Edward Conf.	3 Cunigund
28 William	14 William	4 Adrian
29 Maximilian	15 Hedwig	5 Frederick
30 Wigan	16 Gallus	6 Everard
31 Petronella	17 Etheldreda	7 Perpetua

APPENDIX. 179

JUNE.

BEGINNING.	MIDDLE.	END.
JUNE	**OCTOBER.**	**MARCH.**
1 Nicomede	18 LUKE	8 Phileman
2 Macarius	19 Ptolemy	9 Prudentius
3 Erasmus	20 Wendelia	10 Henrietta
4 Ulrica	21 Ursula	11 Rosina
5 Boniface	22 Corduca	12 Gregory M.
6 Benignus	23 Severus	13 Ernest
7 Lucretia	24 Solomon	14 Zacchary
8 Medard	25 Crispin	15 Isabella
9 Barnimus	26 Amandus	16 Syriac
10 Onuphrius	27 Sabina	17 Patrick
11 BARNABAS	28 SIMON and JUDU	18 Edward
12 Blandina	29 Engelard	19 Joseph
13 Tobias	30 Hartman	20 Rupert
14 Modestus	31 Wolfgang	21 Benedict
	NOVEMBER.	
15 Vitus	1 ALL SAINTS	22 Casimer
16 Justina	2 All Souls	23 Everard
17 Alban	3 Gottlieb	24 Gabriel
18 Paulina	4 Charlotte	25 Annunciation
19 Gervase	5 Eric	26 Emanuel
20 Edward	6 Leonard	27 Hubert
21 Jacobina	7 Erdman	28 Gideon
22 Acharius	8 Claude	29 Eustace
23 Basilius	9 Theodore	30 Guido
24 JOHN BAPTIST	10 Jonas	31 Philip
		APRIL.
25 Elogius	11 Martin	1 Theodore
26 Jeremias	12 Cunibert	2 Theodosia
27 Seven Sleepers	13 Britius	3 Christian
28 Leo	14 Lewin	4 Ambrose
29 PETER and PAUL	15 Machutus	5 Maximus
30 Paul	16 Ottoman	6 Sixtus

JULY.

BEGINNING.	MIDDLE.	END.
JULY.	**NOVEMBER.**	**APRIL.**
1 Theobold	17 Hugh	7 Celestine
2 Visita of Mary	18 Gotschalk	8 Heilman
3 Cornelius	19 Elizabeth	9 Bogislaus
4 Martin	20 Edmund	10 Ezekiel
5 Anselm	21 Presentation	11 Herman
6 Isaiah	22 Cecilia	12 Julius
7 Thim. a Bechet	23 Clement	13 Justin
8 Kilian	24 Lebrecht	14 Tiburtius
9 Cyril	25 Catharine	15 Obadiah
10 Felicity	26 Conrade	16 Carisius
11 Pius	27 Lot	17 Rodolph
12 Henry	28 Gunter	18 Florence
13 Margaret	29 Noah	19 Werner
14 Bonaventure	30 ANDREW	20 Sulpitius
	DECEMBER.	
15 Swithin	1 Arnold	21 Adolphus
16 Enstace	2 Candida	22 Lothario
17 Alexis	3 Cassian	23 GEORGE
18 Caroline	4 Barbara	24 Albert
19 Ruth	5 Abigail	25 MARK
20 Elias	6 Nicholas	26 Raymar
21 Daniel	7 Antonia	27 Anastasius
22 Magdalen	8 Conception	28 Theresa
23 Albertine	9 Joachim	29 Sibylla
24 Christine	10 Judith	30 Joshua
		MAY.
25 JAMES	11 Waldemar	1 PHILIP & JAMES
26 Anne	12 Epimachus	2 Sigismund
27 Berthold	13 Lucy	3 Holy Cross
28 Innocent	14 Israel	4 Florian
29 Martha	15 Johanna	5 Gothard
30 Beatrice	16 Ananias	6 John Evangelist
31 Germain	17 Lazarus	7 Godfrey

AUGUST.

BEGINNING.	MIDDLE.	END.
AUGUST	DECEMBER.	MAY.
1 Peter	18 Christopher	8 Stanislaus
2 Gustavus	19 Manasses	9 Job
3 Augustus	20 Abraham	10 Gordian
4 Perpetua	21 THOMAS	11 Mamertus
5 Dominick	22 Beata	12 Pancratius
6 Transfiguration	23 Ignatius	13 Servatius
7 Donatus	24 Adam and Eve	14 Christiania
8 Ladislaus	25 CHRIST BORN	15 Sophia
9 Romanus	26 STEPHEN	16 Honoratus
10 Lawrence	27 JOHN	17 Pascal
11 Titus	28 INNOCENTS	18 Livorius
12 Clara	29 Jonathan	19 Dunstan
13 Hildebrand	30 David	20 Frances
14 Eusebius	31 Sylvester	21 Prudens
	JANUARY.	
15 Assumption	1 CIRCUMCISION	22 Helena
16 Isaac	2 Abel	23 Desiderius
17 Bertram	3 Enoch	24 Esther
18 Emilia	4 Titus	25 Urban
19 Sebald	5 Simeon	26 Augustine
20 Bernard	6 EPIPHANY	27 Bede
21 Athanasius	7 Melchior	28 William
22 Oswald	8 Lueian	29 Mazimilian
23 Zaccheus	9 Caspar	30 Wigan
24 BARTHOLOMEW	10 Paul Hermit	31 Petronella
		JUNE.
25 Lewis	11 Erhard	1 Nicomede
26 Irenæus	12 Reynold	2 Macarius
27 Gebard	13 Hilarius	3 Erasmus
28 Augustine	14 Felix	4 Ulrica
29 John	15 Habakkuk	5 Bonifacius
30 Benjamin	16 Marcellus	6 Benignus
31 Rebecca	17 Anthony	7 Lucretia

SEPTEMBER.

BEGINNING.	MIDDLE.	END.
SEPTEMBER.	JANUARY.	JUNE.
1 Giles	18 Prisca	8 Medard
2 Rachel	19 Ferdinand	9 Barnimus
3 Mansuetus	20 Fabian	10 Onuphrius
4 Moses	21 Agnes	11 BARNABAS
5 Nathaniel	22 Vincent	12 Blandina
6 Magnus	23 Emerantia	13 Tobias
7 Enurchus	24 Timothy	14 Modestus
8 Mary	25 PAUL	15 Vitus
9 Bruno	26 Polycarp	16 Justina
10 Sosthenes	27 Chrysostom	17 Alban
11 Gerard	28 Charles	18 Paulina
12 Otilia	29 Samuel	19 Gervase
13 Christlieb	30 Adelgunda	20 Edward
14 Exaltation	31 Valerius	21 Jacobina
	FEBRUARY.	
15 Constantia	1 Bridget	22 Acharius
16 Euphemia	2 Purific of Mary	23 Basilius
17 Lambert	3 Blaise	24 JOHN BAPTIST
18 Sigfred	4 Veronica	25 Elogius
19 Jonuarius	5 Agatha	26 Jeremias
20 Frederica	6 Dorothea	27 Seven Sleepers
21 MATTHEW	7 Richard	28 Leo
22 Maurice	8 Solomon	29 PETER and PAUL
23 Joel	9 Apollonia	30 Paul
		JULY.
24 John	10 Renata	1 Theobald
25 Cleophas	11 Euphrosyne	2 Visita of Mary
26 Cyprian	12 Severinus	3 Cornelius
27 Cosmo	13 Benigna	4 Martin
28 Wenzel	14 Valentine	5 Anselm
29 MICHAEL	15 Formosus	6 Isaiah
30 Jerome	16 Juliana	7 Thom. a Becket

OCTOBER.

BEGINNING.	MIDDLE.	END.
OCTOBER.	JANUARY.	JULY.
1 Remigius	17 Constantia	8 Kilian
2 Volrade	18 Concordia	9 Cyril
3 Ewald	19 Susanna	10 Felicity
4 Francis	20 Eucharius	11 Pius
5 Charity	21 Eleanor	12 Henry
6 Faith	22 Peter	13 Margaret
7 Hope	23 Reynard	14 Bonaventura
8 Ephraim	24 MATTHIAS	15 Swithin
9 Denys	25 Victor	16 Eustace
10 Amelia	26 Nestor	17 Alexis
11 Burkard	27 Hector	18 Caroline
12 Erenfried	28 Justus	19 Ruth
	MARCH.	
13 Edward Conf.	1 Albin	20 Elias
14 William	2 Louisa	21 Daniel
15 Hedwig	3 Cunigund	22 Magdalen
16 Gallus	4 Adrian	23 Albertine
17 Etheldreda	5 Frederick	24 Christine
18 LUKE	6 Everhard	25 JAMES
19 Ptolemy	7 Perpetua	26 Anne
20 Wendelia	8 Philemon	27 Berthold
21 Ursula	9 Prudentius	28 Innocent
22 Corduca	10 Henrietta	29 Martha
23 Severus	11 Rosina	30 Beatriue
24 Solomon	12 Gregory, M.	31 Germain
		AUGUST.
25 Crispin	13 Ernest	1 Peter
26 Amandus	14 Zachary	2 Gustavus
27 Sabina	15 Isabella	3 Augustus
28 SIMON and JUDE	16 Syriac	4 Perpetua
29 Engelard	17 Patrick	5 Dominick
30 Hartman	18 Edward	6 Transfiguration
31 Wolfgang	19 Joseph	7 Donatus

NOVEMBER.

BEGINNING.	MIDDLE.	END.
NOVEMBER.	MARCH.	AUGUST.
1 ALL SAINTS	20 Rupert	8 Ladislaus
2 All Souls	21 Benedict	9 Romanus
3 Gottlieb	22 Casimer	10 Lawrenre
4 Charlotte	23 Everard	11 Titus
5 Eric	24 Gabriel	12 Clara
6 Leonard	25 Annunciation	13 Hildebrand
7 Erdmann	26 Emanuel	14 Eusebius
8 Claude	27 Hubert	15 Assumption
9 Theodore	28 Gideon	16 Isaac
10 Jonas	29 Eustace	17 Bertram
11 Martin	30 Guido	18 Emilia
12 Cunibert	31 Philip	19 Sebald
	APRIL.	
13 Britius	1 Theodore	20 Bernard
14 Lewin	2 Theodosia	21 Athanasius
15 Machutus	3 Christian	22 Oswald
16 Ottoman	4 Ambrose	23 Zaccheus
17 Hugh	5 Maximus	24 BARTHOLOMEW
18 Gotschalk	6 Sixtus	25 Lewis
19 Elizabeth	7 Celestine	26 Irenæus
20 Edmund	8 Heilman	27 Gebard
21 Presentation	9 Bogislaus	28 Augustine
22 Cecilia	10 Ezekiel	29 John
23 Clement	11 Herman	30 Benjamin
24 Lebrecht	12 Julius	31 Rebecca
		SEPTEMBER.
25 Catharine	13 Justin	1 Giles
26 Conrad	14 Tiburtius	2 Rachel
27 Lot	15 Obadiah	3 Mansuetus
28 Gunter	16 Carisius	4 Moses
29 Noah	17 Rodolph	5 Nathaniel
30 ANDREW	18 Florenc	6 Magnus

APPENDIX. 185

DECEMBER.

BEGINNING.	MIDDLE.	END.
DECEMBER.	APRIL.	SEPTEMBER.
1 Arnold	19 Werner	7 Enurchus
2 Candida	20 Sulpitius	8 Mary
3 Cassian	21 Adolphus	9 Bruno
4 Barbara	22 Lothario	10 Sosthenes
5 Abigail	23 GEORGE	11 Gerard
6 Nicholas	24 Albert	12 Otilia
7 Antonia	25 MARK	13 Christlieb
8 Conception	26 Raymar	14 Exaltation
9 Joachim	27 Anastasius	15 Constantia
10 Judith	28 Theresa	16 Euphemia
11 Waldemar	29 Sibylla	17 Lambert
12 Epimachus	30 Joshua	18 Sigfried
	MAY.	
13 Lucy	1 PHILIP & JAMES	19 Januarius
14 Israel	2 Sigismund	20 Frederica
15 Johanna	3 Holy Cross	21 MATTHEW
16 Ananias	4 Florian	22 Maurice
17 Lazarus	5 Gothard	23 Joel
18 Christopher	6 John Evangelist	24 John
19 Manasses	7 Godfrey	25 Cleophas
20 Abraham	8 Stanislaus	26 Cyprian
21 THOMAS	9 Job	27 Cosmo
22 Beata	10 Gordian	28 Wenzel
23 Ignatius	11 Mamertus	29 MICHAEL
24 Adam and Eve	12 Pancratius	30 Jerome
		OCTOBER.
25 CHRIST BORN	13 Servatius	1 Remigius
26 STEPHEN	14 Christiana	2 Volrade
27 JOHN	15 Sophia	3 Ewald
28 INNOCENTS	16 Honoratus	4 Francis
29 Jonathan	17 Pascal	5 Charity
30 David	18 Livorius	6 Faith
31 Sylvester	19 Dunstan	7 Hope

INDEX.

A.

	PAGE.
Abortion,	107
Acidity of Stomach,	51
Acids, in Heartburn,	54
Acid, Nitric,	73
" Muriat.,	73
Aconite, in Morning Sickness,	37
" " Toothache,	42
" " Jaundice,	70
" " Piles,	73
" " Rheumatism of Womb,	85
" " Inflammation ",	86
Aethusa Cynapium,	13
Aethusa Cynapium in morning sickness,	37
After-birth, delivery of,	119
After-birth, hemorrhage before, during, and after,	120
After pains,	154
Age, for marriage,	4
Alternations of milk,	145
" " taste, during pregnancy,	30
Alkaline Dyspepsia,	52
Aloes in Jaundice,	70
" Piles,	73
Alumina in Constipation,	60
Ammon. mur. in toothache,	44
Anacardium,	13
Anger, inclination to,	13
Anteversion of the Womb,	92
Antipathies,	13
Antimony in Toothache,	43
Anxiety, about the future,	12
Apis mell,	77
„ in Dropsy of Amnion,	80

	PAGE.
Apocynum in Dropsy of Amnion,	80
Appendix,	173
Argentum nitricum in Menstruation during Pregnancy,	81
Arnica in Toothache,	43
Arsenicum "	44
" in Diarrhœa,	68
" Piles,	73
„ Œdema of Labia,	77
„ False waters,	79
" Dropsy of Amnion,	80
" Menstruation during Pregnancy,	81
Aurum in Menstruation during Pregnancy,	81
Aversion to Meat,	30
" Fish,	32
" Water,	32
" Milk and Butter,	32
" Sweet things,	32
" Vegetables,	32

B.

	PAGE.
Baryta,	12
" in Toothache,	44
Belladonna in Morning Sickness,	37
„ in Toothache,	45
" Jaundice,	70
" Piles,	73
" Inflammation of Womb,	86
Bleeding during Pregnancy,	82
Bofareira,	129
Borax in itching of Vulva,	77
Bovista in Leucorrhœa,	78
Breasts, Pain and Tension of,	107
" Engorgement of,	142

INDEX

Breasts, Inflammation of, ... 143
Bright's Disease, ... 101
Bryonia in Toothache, ... 45
" Constipation, ... 59
" Diarrhœa, ... 68

C

Calendar, Lalies perpetual, ... 174
Calcarea in Toothache, ... 45
Calcarea against Piles, ... 74
Calcarea in Leucorrhœa, ... 78
Camphor in Morning Sickness, .. 36
" Against Spasm of Ureters, ... 76
Causticum in Toothache, ... 46
Cannabis in Incontinence of Urine, ... 76
Contharides " " 76
" Against Spasm of Ureters, ... 76
Cannabis against Spasm of Ureters 76
Cantharides in Menstruation during Pregnancy, ... 81
Capsicum in Constipation, ... 61
" Piles, ... 72
" Incontinence of Urine, 76
Copaiba in Piles, ... 72
Carb-veg. in Toothache, ... 46
Castor Oil Plant in Lactation, .. 129
Chamomilla in Uterine Hemorrhage, .. 82
Chamomilla in Toothache, ... 46
" Jaundice, ... 69
Chills and Trembling, ... 109
China in Toothache, ... 47
China in Diarrhœa, ... 68
" Uterine Hemorrhage, .. 83
Cicuta in Incontinence of Urine, 76
Cicuta, ... 13
Cocculus in Leucorrhœa, ... 78
Cocculus during Pregnancy, ... 81

Colomba in Morning Sickness, .. 35
Colchicum in Toothache, ... 47
Colchicum in Jaundice, ... 70
Conception, ... 6
Constipation, ... 56
Convulsions, ... 104
Contraction of Vulva, ... 114
Convalescence after Parturition, ... 123
Conium, ... 13
" In Morning Sickness, .. 36
" In Incontinence of Urine, 76
Cough, ... 95
Cramps and Pains in Abdomen, Back and Loins, ... 87
Crocus in Menstruation during Pregnancy, ... 81
Crocus in Uterine Hemorrhage, 83
Cuprum, ... 13
" In Morning Sickness, .. 36
Cubebs in Piles, ... 72
Cyclamen in Toothache, ... 47

D.

Delivery, too rapid, ... 114
" of After-birth, ... 119
Depressed Nipples, ... 11 & 139
Digitalis in Salivation, ... 39
Derangement of the Stomach, 110
Desires during Pregnancy, 32 & 28
Diarrhoea, ... 66
Diet during Pregnancy, ... 27
Difficulty of Breathing, ...,.. 95
Digitalis, ... 13
" in œdema of Labia, . . 71
" False waters, ... 79
" Dropsy of Amnion, 80
Dropsy of the Amnion, ... 79
Dropsical Affections, ... 98
Dropsy of the Legs, ... 98
Dulcamara in Diarrhœa, , ... 68
Dying, fear of, ... 15

INDEX.

E.

Engorgement of Breasts, ... 142
Euphorbium of Toothache, ... 47
Excess of Waters, ... 79
Excessive Lactation, ... 169
Exercise during Pregnancy . . . 26
Extra Uterine Pregnancy, ... 118

F.

Fainting, ... 94
Falling of the Womb, ... 89
  „ back of the Womb, . . . 90
. . „ forwards   „ 92
False Waters, ... 78
  „ Labor, ... 109
  „ Pains, ... 88
Fault-finding, ... 13
Feebleness and Slowness of Contraction, ... 111
Ferrum in Morning Sickness, . . 37
Ferrum-aceticum in Constipation, ... 61
Fœtal Turbulence, ... 92
Fluoric-acid in Toothache, . . . 47
Full Bloodedness . . , ... 98

G.

Graphite, ... 13

H.

Hæmorrhoids, ... 70
Headache, ... 96
Hydrocyanic-acid in Morning Sickness, ... 38
Hydrorrhoea, ... 78
Hypochondriasis, ... 98

I.

Ignatia in Constipation, ... 60
  „ Piles, ... 73
Incontinence of Urine, ... 74
Inflammation of Womb, ... 85
  „ Vagina, ... 159

Inflammation of Mucous Membrane of Vagina and Womb 159
  „ Asthenic, of Vagina 160
  „ Cavity of neck of Womb 161
  „ Fibrous Structure of Womb 161
  „ Peritoneum, ... 162
  „ Sub-Peritoneal tissue, 165
  „ Post-Partem, 158 to 169
  „ Veins of Womb, . . . 167
  , Crural and Pelvic Veins, ... 168
Iodine in Salivation, ... 39
Inversion of the Womb, ... 122
Ipecae in Morning Sickness . . . 37
  „ Uterine Hemorrhage, . . 82
Irritability of Womb, ... 85
Irregularity of Pains, ... 113
Itching of the Vulva, ... 77
Jaundice, ... 69

K.

Kali-bichrom, in Constipation, 61
Kiesteine, ... 14
Kreosote in Morning Sickness 35
  „ Toothache, ... 48

L.

Lactation, ... 126
  „ Excessive, ... 169
Ladies Perpetual Calendar . . . 174
Laurocerasus, ... 13
Ledum, ... 13
Leucorrhoea, ... 77
Liver Spots, ... 69
Lochial Discharge, ... 156
Lochia, suppression of, ... 158
Lobelia, ... 13
Lycopodium in Constipation, . . 60

M.

	PAGE
Magnesia in Toothache,	48
Marriage,	1
Menstruation during Pregnancy,	80
Mercurius in Salivation,	39
,, Toothache,	48
,, Jaundice,	69
Mezereum in Toothache,	48
Milk-Fever,	126
,, ,,	142
,, Alterations of	145
,, Healthy standard of,	145
,, Colostrum of,	146
,, Age of Nurse,	146
,, Age of	147
,, Constitution of Nurse,	148
,, Influence of Pregnancy,	148
,, ,, Menstruation,	148
,, ,, Complexion,	149
,, ,, Food,	149
,, ,, Quantity	149
,, ,, Acute Fevers,	149
,, ,, Moral Emotions	149
,, ,, Chronic disease	150
,, ,, Consumption,	150
,, Quantity of Sugar in,	151
,, ,, Casein,	151
,, ,, Butter	151
,, Comparison with Cow's	151
,, Incontinence of,	153
Milk Leg,	168
Millefolium against Bleeding Piles,	73
Moles,	117
Morning Sickness,	33
Moschus in Constipation,	61

N.

Nervousness,	111
Nipples, Soreness of,	137
,, Depressed,	139
Nitric-acid,	13
,, in Salivation,	39
Nux,	13

	PAGE
Nux in Toothache,	49
,, Dyspepsia,	53
,, Heartburn,	53
,, Constipation, 59 to	60
,, Jaundice,	69
,, Piles,	73
,, Retention of Urine,	75
,, Inflammation of Womb,	86
,, In Morning Sickness,	35

O.

Obliquity of the Orifice,	116
Œdema of the Labia,	116
,, ,,	115
Opium in Constipation,	60
,, Itching of Vulva,	77
Ox-gall in Constipation,	62

P.

Pains and Cramps of the Stomach,	55
Pain and Tension of Breasts,	107
Pains, Relaxation of,	113
,, Suspension of,	113
,, Irregularity of	113
Palpitation of the Heart,	95
Parturition, Convalescence after	123
Perpetual Calendar, Ladies,	174
Piles,	70
Phosphorus in Diarrhœa,	68
Phosphor in Acidity,	53
Platina in Constipation,	60
,, Uterine Hemorrhage,	82
Plethora,	98
Plumbum in Constipation,	61
Post-Partem Inflammations,	158
Pregnancy,	7
,, extra-uterine,	118
,, duration of,	8
,, state of Breasts in,	11
,, state of Urine	13
,, management of,	15
,, treatment of,	22
,, superstitions about,	24

INDEX.

	PAGE.
Pregnancy, exercise in,	26
„ diet during,	27
„ perverted tastes during	30
„ menstruation during,	80
Puerperal Mania,	169
Pulsatilla in Salivation,	39
„ Leucorrhoea,	78
„ Toothache,	49
„ Diarrhœa,	67
„ Piles',	72
„ Acidity,	53

R

Relaxation of Pains,	113
Retention of Urine,	75
Retroversion of the Womb,	90
Rheumatism of Womb	83
Rhododendron in Toothache,	49
Rhus in Toothache,	49
„ Diarrhœa,	68
„ Incontinence of Urine,	76
Rigidity and Laxity of Abdomen,	88
„ of the Neck of Womb,	116
„ of Vulva	114

S.

Sabina in Toothache,	50
„ Jaundice,	70
„ Piles,	73
„ Uterine Hemorrhage,	83
Salivation,	38
Scilla in Dropsy of Amnion	80
Secale in Morning Sickness,	36
„ Toothache,	50
„ Diarrhœa,	67
„ Uterine Hemorrhage,	83
Sepia in Morning Sickness,	36
„ Toothache,	50
„ Itching of Vulva,	77
„ Leucorrhœa,	78
Silex in Toothache,	50
Sleeplessness,	96
Slowness and Feebleness of Contions	111

	PAGE.
Sore Nipples	137
Spasm of the Ureters,	76
Spasm and Inflammation of Womb,	86
Spitting of Blood,	96
Spigelia,	13
„ in Toothache,	50
Staphysagria in Toothache,	50
Stramonium in Piles,	73
Sulphur in Morning Sickness,	38
„ Salivation,	39
„ Toothache,	51
Sulphuric-acid in Acidity,	53
Sulphur in Acidity,	53
„ Constipation,	59
„ Diarrhœa,	68
„ Jaundice,	69
„ Piles,	73
„ Leucorrhœa,	78
„ Itching of Vulva,	77
Suspension of Pains,	113
Swelling of Anterior Lip,	117

T

Tabacum in Morning Sickness	36
Thrombus,	115
Toothache,	40
Trembling and Chills,	109

V.

Varicose Veins,	106
Veratrum in Morning Sickness	36
„ Salivation,	39
„ Constipation,	62

W.

Waters, excess of,	79
„ False,	78
Weaning,	170
White Weakness,	77
Womb, Changes of, after Parturition,	153

Z.

Zincum in Morning Sickness,	36
„ Constipation,	62